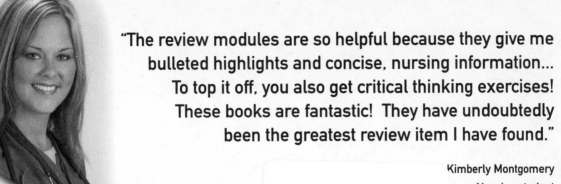

"The review modules are so helpful because they give me bulleted highlights and concise, nursing information... To top it off, you also get critical thinking exercises! These books are fantastic! They have undoubtedly been the greatest review item I have found."

Kimberly Montgomery
Nursing student

Terim Richards *Nursing student*

"I immediately went to my nurse manager after I failed the NCLEX® and she referred me to ATI. I was able to discover the areas I was weak in, and focused on those areas in the review modules and online assessments. I was much more prepared the second time around!"

Molly Obetz *Nursing student*

"The ATI review books were very helpful in preparing me for the NCLEX®. I really utilized the review summaries and the critical thinking exercises at the end of each chapter. It was nice to review the key points in the areas I was weak in and not have to read the entire book."

Lindsey Koeble *Nursing student*

"I attribute my success totally to ATI. That is the one thing I used between my first and second attempt at the NCLEX®....with ATI I passed!"

Danielle Platt *Nurse Manager • Children's Mercy Hospital • Kansas City, MO*

"The year our hospital did not use the ATI program, we experienced a 15% decrease in the NCLEX® pass rates. We reinstated the ATI program the following year and had a 90% success rate."

"As a manager, I have witnessed graduate nurses fail the NCLEX® and the devastating effects it has on their morale. Once the nurses started using ATI, it was amazing to see the confidence they had in themselves and their ability to go forward and take the NCLEX® exam."

Mary Moss *Associate Dean of Nursing and Health Programs • Mid-State Technical College • Rapids, WI*

"I like that ATI lets students know what to expect from the NCLEX®, helps them plan their study time and tells them what to do in the days and weeks before the exam. It is different from most of the NCLEX® review books on the market."

Contributors

Penny Fauber-Moore, RN, MS

Director, School of Practical Nursing
Stonewall Jackson School of Practical Nursing
Lexington, Virginia

Sue Kilgore, RN, BSN

Park University
Parkville, Missouri
Shawnee Mission Medical Center

Editor

Leslie Schaaf Treas, RN, PhD(c), MSN, CNNP

Director of Research and Development
Assessment Technologies Institute™, LLC
Overland Park, Kansas

Copyright Notice

Important Notice to the Reader of this Publication

Assessment Technologies Institute, LLC is the publisher of this publication. The publisher reserves the right to modify, change, or update the content of this publication at any time. The content of this publication, such as text, graphics, images, information obtained from the publisher's licensors, and other material contained in this publication are for informational purposes only. The content is not providing medical advice, and is not intended to be a substitute for professional medical advice, diagnosis, or treatment. Always seek the advice of your primary care provider or other qualified health provider with any questions you may have regarding a medical condition. Never disregard professional medical advice or delay in seeking it because of something you have read in this publication. If you think you may have a medical emergency, call your primary care provider or 911 immediately.

The publisher does not recommend or endorse any specific tests, primary care providers, products, procedures, processes, opinions, or other information that may be mentioned in this publication. Reliance on any information provided by the publisher, the publisher's employees, or others contributing to the content at the invitation of the publisher, is solely at your own risk. Healthcare professionals need to use their own clinical judgment in interpreting the content of this publication, and details such as medications, dosages or laboratory tests and results should always be confirmed with other resources.†

This publication may contain health or medical-related materials that are sexually explicit. If you find these materials offensive, you may not want to use this publication.

The publishers, editors, advisors, and reviewers make no representations or warranties of any kind or nature, including but not limited to the accuracy, reliability, completeness, currentness, timeliness, or the warranties of fitness for a particular purpose or merchantability, nor are any such representations implied with respect to the content herein (with such content to include text and graphics), and the publishers, editors, advisors, and reviewers take no responsibility with respect to such content. The publishers, editors, advisors, and reviewers shall not be liable for any actual, incidental, special, consequential, punitive or exemplary damages (or any other type of damages) resulting, in whole or in part, from the reader's use of, or reliance upon, such content.

Introduction to Assessment–Driven Review

To prepare candidates for the licensure exam, many different methods have been used. Assessment Technologies Institute™, LLC, (ATI) offers Assessment–Driven Review™ (ADR), a newer approach for customized board review based on candidate performance on a series of content-based assessments.

The ADR method is a four-part process that serves as a type of competency-assessment for preparation for the NCLEX®. The goal is to increase preparedness and subsequent pass rate on the licensure exam. Used as a comprehensive program, the ADR is designed to help learners focus their review and remediation efforts, thereby increasing their confidence and familiarity with the NCLEX® content. This type of program identifies learners at risk for failure in the early stages of nursing education and provides a path for prescriptive learning prior to the licensure examination.

The ADR approach may be preferable to a traditional "crash course" style of review for a variety of reasons. Time restriction is a fundamental barrier to comprehensive review.

Because of the difficulty in keeping up with the expansiveness of information available today, a more efficient and directed approach is needed. Individualized review that starts with the areas of deficit helps the learner narrow the focus and begin customized remediation instead of a blanket A-to-Z approach. Additionally, review that occurs sequentially over time may be preferable to after-the-fact efforts after completion of a program when faculty are no longer available to assist with remediation.

Early identification of content weaknesses may prove advantageous to progressive program success. "Smaller bites" for content achievement and a shortened lapse of time between the introduction of course content and remediation efforts is likely to be more effective in catching the struggling learner before it is too late. Regular feedback keeps learners "on track" and reduce attrition rate by identifying the learner who is "slipping." This approach provides the opportunity to tutor or implement intensified instruction before the learner reaches a point of no return and drops out of the program.

Step I: Proctored Assessment

The ADR program is a method using a prescriptive learning strategy that begins with a proctored, diagnostic assessment of the learner's mastery of nursing content. The topics covered within the ADR program are based on the current NCLEX® Test Plan. Proctored assessments are administered in paper-pencil and online formats. Scores are reported instantly with Internet testing or within 24 hours for paper-pencil testing. Individual performance profiles list areas of deficiencies and guide the learner's review and remediation of the missed topics. This road map serves as a starting point for self-directed study for NCLEX® success. Learners receive a cumulative Report Card showing scores from all assessments taken throughout the program—beginning to end. Like reading a transcript, the learner and educator can monitor the sequential progress, step-by-step, an assessment at a time

Step II: Modular Reviews

A good test is one that supports teaching and learning. The score report identifies areas of content mastery as well as a means for correction and improvement of weak content areas. Eight review modules contain concise summaries of topics with a clinical overview, therapeutic nursing management, and client teaching. Key concepts are provided to streamline the study process. The ATI modules are not intended to serve as a primary teaching source. Instead, they are designed to summarize the material relevant to the licensure exam and entry-level practice.

Learners are taught to integrate holistic care with a critical thinking approach into the review material to promote clinical application of course content. The learner constructs responses to open-ended questions to stimulate higher-order thinking. The learner may provide rationales for actions in various clinical scenarios and generate explanations of why the solution may be effective in similar clinical situations. These exercises serve as the venue to shift from traditional didactic memorization of facts toward the use of analytical and evaluative reason in a client-related situation. The clinical application scenarios involve the learner actively in the problem-solving process and stimulate an attitude of inquiry.

These exercises are designed to provoke creative problem solving for the individual learner as well as collaborative dialogue for groups of learners in the classroom. Through group discussion, learners discover the technique of elaboration. Learners use group dialogue to increase their understanding of nursing content. In study groups, they may pose questions to their peers or explain various topics in their own words, adding personal experiences with clients and examples from previously acquired knowledge of the topic. Together they learn to reframe problems and assemble evidence to support conclusions. Through the integration of multiple perspectives and the synergy involved in the exchange of ideas, this approach may also facilitate the development of effective working relationships and patterns for lifelong learning. Critical thinking exercises for each topic area situate instruction into a problem-solving environment that can capture learners' attention, increase motivation to learn, and frame the content into an application context. Additionally, the group involvement can model the process for effective team interaction.

Step III: Non-Proctored Assessments

The third step is the use of online assessments that allow users to test from any site with an Internet connection. This online battery identifies specific areas of content weakness for further directed study. The interactive style provides the learner with immediate feedback on all response options. Rationales provide additional information about the correctness of an answer to supplement learners' understanding of the concept. Detailed explanations are provided for each incorrect response to clarify topics that learners often confuse, misunderstand, or fail to remember. Readiness to learn is often peaked when errors are uncovered; thus, immediate feedback is provided when learners are most motivated to find the answer. A Performance Profile summarizes learners' mastery of content. Question descriptors for each missed item are used to stimulate inquiry and further exploration of the topic. The online assessment is intended to extend the learners' preparation for NCLEX® in a way that is personally suited to their deficiencies.

Step IV: ATI-PLAN™ DVD Series

This multi-disk set contains more than 28 hours of nursing review material. The DVD content is designed to complement ATI's Content Mastery SeriesTM review modules and online assessments. Using the ATI-PLAN™ navigational points, learners can easily find the content areas they want to review.

Recognizing that individuals process information in a variety of ways, ATI developed the ATI-PLAN™ DVD series to offer nursing review in a way that simulates the classroom. However, individuals viewing the ATI-PLAN™ DVDs can navigate through more than 28 hours of material to their topics of choice. Nursing review is available at the convenience of the learner and can be replayed as often as necessary to ensure mastery of content.

The regulation of personal learning goals and the ability to plan and pursue academic intentions are the keys to successful learning. The expert teacher is the one who can determine individual learning needs and appropriate strategies to master learning. The ADR program is an efficient method of helping students prepare for the nursing licensure exam using frequent and systematic content review directed by the identified areas of content weakness. The interactive approach for mastery of nursing content focused in the areas of greatest need is likely to increase student success on the licensure exam.

ATI's ADR method parallels the nursing process in concept and in design. Both provide a framework for solving actual and potential problems purposefully and methodically. Assessment ADR-style is accomplished with ATI's battery of proctored assessments. Diagnosis is facilitated by the individual and group score reports the proctored assessments generate. Planning for improving performance in identified areas of weakness incorporates ATI's modular review system. Implementation begins with modular review and culminates in use of ATI's online assessments to validate improvement. Evaluation is reflected in the score reports, and performance can then be strengthened or further improved with the ATI-PLAN™ DVD series. Just like the nursing process, ATI's ADR prescriptive learning method often leads to specific, measurable results and highly desirable outcomes.

Table of Contents

Individual and Community

Key Points

- Wellness is a lifestyle that enhances each of the five dimensions of health, including nutrition.
- Food has three basic functions: provide energy sources, build tissues, and regulate metabolic processes.
- Nutrients are delivered to the body through the processes of ingestion, absorption, digestion, energy production, and excretion.
- Nutrients provide three essential functions:
  - Providing energy
  - Facilitating growth, development, and maintenance
  - Prevention of disease and bodily dysfunction
- Good nutrition means a person receives and uses substances obtained from a varied diet.
- Dietary guidelines are based on a concern about chronic health problems in an aging population.
- Factors affecting nutrition: age, lifestyle, food preferences, ethnicity, culture, religion, and economics.
- *Healthy People 2010* is focused on health promotion and disease prevention. The Internet link for the Healthy People program is: http://www.health.gov/healthypeople.

Overview

Health is defined as the absence of disease; however, it must include broad attention to basic human needs and focus on each of the five dimensions of health, including nutrition. Nutrition is the science of food and nutrients, their action and interaction, in relation to providing the body with the necessary substances to maintain homeostasis. Nutritional balance impacts health maintenance and disease prevention and is essential for growth and optimal bodily function. The process for nutrient use by the body includes: ingestion, absorption, digestion, energy production, and excretion.

Role of Nutrition in Health Promotion

Nutrition is the study of nutrients and the processes by which they are used by the body. The primary role of nutrients is to provide the building blocks for the functioning and maintenance of the body. Nutrition is the mainstay of each health dimension.

Physical and Psychological Dimensions of Health

- **Physical**: Efficiency of the body to function appropriately and meet daily energy requirements
- **Intellectual**: Use of cognitive abilities to learn and adapt to changes in the environment
- **Emotional**: Capacity to express feelings appropriately
- **Social**: Ability to interact with people in an acceptable manner
- **Spiritual**: Cultural beliefs that give purpose to human existence

Assessment of Nutritional Status

Nutritional assessment is the process of determining the nutritional status of an individual and the nutritional deficiencies affecting health and wellness. An assessment of the dietary intake and the body's utilization of nutrients is essential to designing a nutritional plan for growth and health maintenance.

- **Clinical examination** by a primary health care provider, nurse, or dietitian to note signs of nutritional health, such as distribution of fat (upper-body or lower-body obesity); appearance of skin, hair, nails, teeth, and wounds or lesions.
- It is important to collect data on the food a person eats for a 24-hour period through a **food record** and a **diet history**.
- Family tree
- Biochemical analysis of samples of body tissues, such as blood and urine tests, to see how the body uses nutrients
- **Anthropometric measurements** such as height, weight, and limb circumference
- **Skin-fold thickness** using skin calipers or other tools
- **Weight-for-Height tables**: Estimating body weight using the Metropolitan Life Insurance Company Weight-for-Height tables is one common way to determine a person's desired weight based on sex and body-frame size.
- **Body mass index (BMI)**: More recently in the health-related literature determinations of healthy weight are based on body mass index (BMI). The nurse may calculate BMI by:

$$\underline{\text{Body weight (kg)}} \qquad \text{or} \qquad \underline{\text{Body weight (lb) x 703.1}}$$
$$\text{Height}^2 \text{ (meters)} \qquad\qquad\qquad \text{Height}^2 \text{ (inches)}$$

BMI charts list specific parameters for weight-for-height indices. Generally, when the BMI exceeds 25, health risks increase. A healthy range is 18.5-24.9 for most people. A moderately overweight person typically has a BMI of 25-29; obesity is marked by BMI of 30+ and 40+ is considered morbid obesity.

- **Underwater weighing**: Method for estimating total body fat: weighing a person on a standard scale and then again submerged in water. The difference between the two measurements is an estimation of body fat.

- **Bioelectrical impedance**: Method that uses low-energy electrical current. The more fat a person has, the more impedance to an electrical flow will occur.
- **Infrared light to bicep**: Used to assess the fat composition in proportion to muscle
- **Dual x-ray photon absorptiometry** (DEXA): X-ray system that separates body weight into fat, fat-free soft tissue, and bone

Overnutrition

- Obesity is a state in which nutritional intake exceeds the body's need.
- U.S. citizens generally consume more saturated fats than are needed. This contributes to many disease processes.
- Effects of obesity:
  - Social
    - Cultural desirability for thinness
    - Leanness associated with attractiveness
    - Prejudice and discriminatory practices with selection and promotion decisions.
  - Psychological
    - Body image disturbances
    - Eating disorders
  - Medical
    - Shortened life expectancy
    - Increased risk of diabetes, heart disease and hypertension, joint dysfunction, gall bladder disease, colorectal cancer and breast cancer, lung-function impairment, and endocrine abnormalities

Malnutrition

- Due to imbalanced nutrient and energy needs
- May be caused either by intake of too few nutrients or excessive consumption of nutrient- poor foods
- An obese person may suffer from malnutrition.
- Other populations at risk for malnutrition include young children, adolescents, low-income persons, the elderly, hospitalized clients, and chronic alcohol users.

Dietary Guidelines

- Eat a variety of foods.
- Maintain healthy weight.
- Choose a diet low in saturated fat and cholesterol.
- Choose a diet with plenty of vegetables, fruits, and grain products.
- Use sugar only in moderation.
- Use salt sparingly, particularly if health status warrants dietary restriction.
- Drink alcohol in moderation.

The Food Guide Pyramid

The four basic food groups guide was developed by the United States Department of Agriculture as a general guideline for planning a diet that is well-balanced for persons older than age 2. The most current edition of this guide now includes five basic food groups and is known as the Food Guide Pyramid. The recommended daily intake of each group, based on the Pyramid, follows:

- **Breads, cereals, rice, and pasta**: 6-11 servings per day
- **Vegetables**: 3-5 servings; **Fruit**: 2-4 servings
- **Milk, yogurt, and cheese**: 2-3 servings
- **Meat, poultry, fish, dry beans, eggs, and nuts**: 2-3 servings
- **Fats, oils, and sweets**: Use sparingly
- **Calories**: The average middle-aged male needs 2200-2500 kcal/day. The average middle-aged female requires approximately 1800 kcal/day. Extra calories are stored as fat or must be burned by activity.

The major change in the recommended daily allowances has been the emphasis on breads and cereals, fruits, and vegetables. This was done to provide the bulk of dietary energy from carbohydrates, while limiting fat intake.

Food, Energy, and Nutrients

Energy-yielding nutrients provide different amounts of energy. Carbohydrates (CHO) and proteins each provide 4 kcal/gram. Fats contain 9 kcal/gram. Alcohol contains 7 kcal/gram and is not considered a nutrient.

Carbohydrates

- The primary function of CHO is to provide the body with energy.
- Carbohydrates are composed of carbon, hydrogen, and oxygen (CHO).
- They consist of simple CHO called sugars, and include sucrose, glucose, dextrose, and fructose.
- Complex CHO includes starches and fibers.
- Dietary fiber is the substance in plant foods that are not digested by the body. Fiber adds bulk to the feces and will stimulate peristalsis to make elimination easier.
- Glucose provides the most efficient form of energy.
- Provide 4 kcal/gram of energy

Proteins

- Proteins provide 4.5 kcal/gm of energy.
- Functions include roles in the structure of bones, muscles, enzymes, hormones, blood, and the immune system.
- Formed by linking amino acids in various combinations
- Like carbohydrates and fats, proteins are comprised of carbon, oxygen, and hydrogen atoms and are formed by the linking of amino acids.

Fats

- Lipids are the densest form of energy available and produce 9 kcal/gm of energy.

- Lipids, which are fats and oils, are composed of the elements: carbon, hydrogen, and a few oxygen atoms.
- Lipids are insoluble in water but dissolve in certain organic solvents.
- Triglycerides are the primary form of fat in food.
- Generally speaking, oils are lipids that are liquid at room temperature, and fats are solids at room temperature.
- Fats are generally divided into three categories: triglycerides, phospholipids, and sterols.
- Fats serve as a component of all cell structures; they have a role in hormone production and provide padding to protect vital organs.
- Plant oils tend to contain many unsaturated fatty acids.

Vitamins

- The main function of vitamins is to enable chemical reactions in the body.
- Vitamins yield no usable energy for the body.
- Vitamin compounds function to indirectly assist other nutrients to meet bodily needs.
- Each of the thirteen essential vitamins has a special function. The human body needs thirteen and each has a special function.
- Two classes of vitamins:
  - Water-soluble: C and B complex
  - Fat-soluble: A, E, D, and K
- Eating a variety of foods is the best way to consume sufficient vitamin intake. Dietary forms are more biologically available than multivitamin tablets.

Minerals

- Minerals serve structural purposes and are found in all body fluids and tissues.
- Sixteen essential minerals are divided into two categories: major and trace.
- Minerals are plentiful in all foods, although some may be lost in food processing.
- Organic minerals are structurally simple compounds and contain the carbon-hydrogen bond.
- Inorganic minerals exist as groups of atom-lacking carbon bound with hydrogen.

Water

- Water provides a means of transportation for nutrients.
- Water acts as a solvent and a lubricant.
- It is the by-product of metabolism.
- The human body is approximately 60% water.
- Need to consume the equivalent of 2 liters of fluid/day from foods and beverages (approximately 8 cups). Foods with a high water content include melons, cantaloupe, and berries.

Calculating the Energy Content in Food

To determine caloric expenditure available in a carbohydrate, start by multiplying the amount of CHO (gm) X 4 grams: 35 grams X 4 kcal/gram = 140 kcal. Fat composition is calculated by multiplying the total fat content of the food X 9: 30 grams X 9 kcal/gram = 270 kcal. And protein energy is produced in the amount determined by: 25 grams X 4.5 kcal/gram = 112.5 kcal.

To figure out the percentage energy (kcal) as carbohydrate, fat, or protein that is consumed in a day, obtain the total amount of CHO, fat or protein (grams) per day and multiply times the kcal of energy it produces. In this example, carbohydrate 140 kcal, fat 270 kcal, and protein 112.5 kcal = 522.5. Then divide by the total caloric intake that day. To exemplify the point, based on calculations on an 1800 kcal/day diet.

> % of kcal as carbohydrate: 140 ÷ 1800 = 7.8%
>
> % of kcal as fat: 270 ÷ 1800 = 15.0%
>
> % of kcal as protein: 112.5 ÷ 1800 = 6.2%

Healthy Weight Management

Nurses play a vital role in fostering healthy living habits by teaching clients the basics for good nutrition. Some general recommendations for health promotion and disease prevention include:

Diet

- Eat a well-balanced diet to prevent:
  - Birth anomalies and low birthweight in infants
  - Impaired growth in infants and children
  - Poor resistance to infection and disease throughout the lifespan
  - Deficiency diseases, such as scurvy, pellagra, iron-deficiency anemia, rickets, osteoporosis
- Take in sufficient amounts of calcium to facilitate bone and teeth mineralization in children and prevent osteoporosis in adults.
- Consume recommended amounts of fluoride to strengthen tooth enamel and prevent dental caries.
- Include enough dietary fiber to promote bowel regularity.
- Moderate the amount of fat intake to recommended ratios for total, saturated, unsaturated fats, and cholesterol to reduce the risk of coronary artery disease.
- Limit caloric intake to maintain a desired weight for age, sex, and body frame.
- Avoid taking high doses of fat-soluble vitamins to prevent toxicities.
- Reduce sodium intake to lessen the risk of or symptoms related to hypertension, Ménière's disease, and kidney problems in susceptible persons.
- Moderate the portion size to prevent overeating.
- Consume adequate amounts of potassium because of the link to stroke.

Physical Activity

- Regular, vigorous activity is recommended for a minimum of 30 minutes/day at least three times a week to strengthen cardiovascular condition.

- Loss in bone density is related to lack of weight-bearing exercise.
- Heart attack risk is greater in the person with a sedentary lifestyle.
- The risk of obesity exponentially increases with lack of exercise.

Lifestyle

- Limit alcohol intake to a maximum of two drinks per day no more than 1-2 times per week.
- Chronic alcohol use can cause cirrhosis, premature aging, fetal alcohol syndrome, and increase the risk for accidents.

Nutritional History

Healthy weight control means stable body weight within the recommended range for sex, height, age, and frame. Little fluctuation from the ideal weight is optimal for health maintenance. The nurse assessing the nutritional status may ask questions about dietary patterns and healthy weight control.

- What is your baseline weight?
- What is the lowest weight that you had this past year?
- What is the most that you have weighed this past year?
- What is the largest and smallest clothing size that you are happy with? Are you content with your current weight and appearance?
- What weight are you able to maintain without feeling hungry?
- Are you taking medication to increase or suppress your appetite, increase metabolism, or alter fat absorption from food?
- Are you on medication that alters the taste of food?
- Do you take medication for mood or sleep?
- Do you smoke? How often?
- Do you consume alcohol? How often? How much?
- Do you exercise? How often? How long? How vigorous? Why?
- How many times in this last year have you observed a weight reduction diet? Or a diet to gain weight?
- Do you have a past or present history of anorexia nervosa or bulimia nervosa?
- Do you tend to snack? When? Why?
- Are members of your family obese or underweight?
- Do you have dietary restrictions related to religion, culture, or family influences?
- Do you have enough money to buy the type and amount of food that you would like to eat?
- Are you healthy now? Do you have a past history of any health disorder that affected your appetite?
- What is your basic body shape? When you gain weight, where does fat typically deposit?

Excess Body Mass

- Body mass above a population's weight-for-height standard, usually 10-20% above the healthy body weight.
- Obesity is the relative excess amount of fat in the total body composition; usually a body fat content above 24% in males and above 33% in females is considered obese.
- There are individual variations in a person's weight, depending on age, body shape, metabolic rate, genetic makeup, gender, and physical activity.
- Some body fat is essential. Males need at least 3% for survival and females about 12% for menstruation.
- Obesity is linked to Type 2 diabetes and hypertension, coronary artery disease, and peripheral vascular disease.
- Dietary principles should be based on five characteristics:
  - Realistic goals
  - Caloric intake in diet adjusted to bodily need
  - Nutritional adequacy
  - Culturally desirable
  - Caloric intake balance to maintain weight
- A sensible food plan should include carbohydrate as 55% of total calories, protein as 15% of total calories, and fats about 30% of total calories.
- Satiety is influenced by complex and interacting factors:
  - Factors that influence hunger
    - Central nervous system: hypothalamus
    - Bodily organs: stomach, small intestine, liver, hormones (endorphins, serotonin, insulin, sex hormones), digestive enzymes
    - Disease states: obesity, anorexia nervosa, cancer, reflux, ulcer disease, AIDS
    - Emotional factors: stress, mood
    - Environmental factors: weather, humidity
  - Factors that influence appetite
    - Lifestyle: personal eating habits, preferences, daily schedule and pace
    - Social influences: cultural influences, religious restrictions
    - Learned preferences and aversions: past and present experience with food, tastes, food association with place, time, event, or person
    - Pleasurable factors: palatability, taste, texture, odor, presentation
    - Medication effects: appetite stimulants, appetite depressants, medications that change the flavor (metallic), sedatives
    - Disease states: cancer
    - Metabolic factors: genetic, basal metabolic rate, neurotransmitter levels, insulin regulation
- Dietary fiber can provide a feeling of fullness, and thus, curb the tendency to overeat.

Reduced Body Mass

A person who is more than 10% below the average weight for height and age is considered underweight. Serious consequences occur in people who are 20% under desired weight, including decreased resistance to infection and poor general health.

- Causes include wasting diseases, inadequate food intake, malabsorption, hormonal imbalances, and energy imbalances.
- Dietary treatment includes a high-calorie diet at least 50% above standard, high protein to rebuild tissues, high CHO to provide energy, moderate fat to add calories, and good sources of vitamins and minerals.
- A variety of foods, if served attractively, increase appetite and the desire to eat more. Nutritious, calorie-rich snacks are included throughout the day.

Consumer Food Decision Making

- Food selection patterns depend on taste, as well as price, product safety, nutrition, ease of preparation, and food preparation time.
- Overall, total fruit and vegetable consumption is increasing because dietary guidelines recommend an increased number of servings.
- Having cereal products at the base of the Food Guide Pyramid makes it likely that consumption of cereal-based foods will increase.
- Beef consumption has decreased, while poultry and fish consumptionhave increased.
- The consumption of dairy products has increased, especially the low-fat variety.
- Effective food-buying styles are important and include knowing the food budget, lifestyles of family members, care of any special needs, how often shopping is done, and where shopping takes place.

Food Labeling

- Food labeling in the U.S. is based on standards set by the 1990 Nutrition Labeling and Education Act.
- Nutrition facts are reflected on percent of daily values of a 2000 kcal/diet.
- Reference daily intakes (RDIs) set standards for protein, vitamins, and minerals based on current **U.S. recommended daily allowances (RDAs)**. RDAs are recommended intakes of nutrients that are sufficient to meet the needs of most (97%) healthy individuals of similar age and gender.
- **Daily reference values (DRVs)** are for nutrients, for which there are no specific RDAs or a related nutritional standard.
- Food labels must specify the percent of each of the following: total food energy (kilocalories), food energy from fat, total fat, saturated fat, cholesterol, sodium, total carbohydrate, dietary fiber, sugars, protein, vitamin C, calcium, and iron.

Food Additives

Chemicals can be intentionally added to foods for the following reasons:

- Enriching foods with added nutrients
- Producing uniform qualities (color, flavor, aroma, texture, and general appearance)

- Standardizing functional factors (thickening or stabilization)
- Preserving foods to prevent oxidation and destruction of food components by metals and other substances
- Controlling acidity or alkalinity to improve flavor and texture

The Delaney Clause is the 1958 Food Additives Amendment to the Federal Food, Drug, and Cosmetic Act of 1938 that bans any intentional food additive found to induce cancer in man or animal.

Food Quality and Safety

- Food safety is a concern in today's society. It is an expectation that governmental agencies will supervise the production and preparation of food to ensure safety.
- The FDA (Food and Drug Administration) is the law-enforcement agency responsible for ensuring that the food supply is safe, pure, and wholesome.
- The agency enforces rules and regulations that control the following:
  - Food sanitation and quality control
  - Chemical contaminants and pesticides
  - Food additives
  - Regulating the movement of food across state lines
  - Maintaining the nutrition labeling of food
  - Ensuring the safety of public food service
  - Ensuring the safety of meat and milk
- Food safety and quality are also accomplished through consumer education and general public information. Running the water from a home tap for 30 seconds prior to using the water may reduce the amount of lead content in the water.
- The majority of environmental contaminants that are found in foods are fat-soluble. The best way to minimize the exposure is to trim all excess fat off of meats and peel, wash, or discard the skin.
- Toxic elements in foods, such as certain types of mushrooms, raw fish, and raw egg whites, are eliminated with thorough cooking.
- Contamination with pathogenic organisms to food or water, transmission through cross- contamination via handling food, or feces can cause food-borne illness. Primary measures to control exposure to unhealthy bacterial growth involve proper food handling, preparation, and storage practices. Strict hand washing is highly effective in preventing the spread of food-borne illness.

Impact of Culture on Diet

Personal habits regarding food develop as part of our social and cultural background, as well as our lifestyle. All of our food habits are related to our way of life, our values, beliefs, and individual situations.

Characteristics of Ethnic Diets

- Food habits develop from personal, cultural, social, economic, and psychological influences.

- Many foods in our culture take on symbolic meaning related to major life experiences.
- Since ancient times, ceremonies and religious rites involving food have been important.

Food Preferences and Preparations

Preferences and preparation vary among cultural groups and many are based on religious customs. Examples follow:

- **Jewish Orthodox**: Basic dietary law is the "Rules of Kashruth." Foods selected and prepared are called kosher.
    - No pork is allowed; meat is cleansed of all blood.
    - Combining of meat and milk is not permitted.
    - Only fish with fins and scales are allowed.
    - No eggs with a blood spot are used.
    - Representative foods include bagels, blintzes, knishes, lox, and matzo
- **Mexican**: Follow food habits of early Spanish settlers and Native Americans.
    - Dried beans, chili peppers, and corn are staple items.
    - Small amounts of meat and eggs are eaten.
    - Some fruits are consumed depending on availability.
    - Coffee is main beverage.
    - Representative foods include tortillas and rice.
- **Asian/Chinese/Japanese**: Believe that refrigeration diminishes flavor; use fresh foods and cook quickly.
    - Woks are used for cooking.
    - Vegetables are usually served crisp.
    - Meats are used in small amounts and in combined dishes.
    - Fresh fruits are eaten often.
    - Rice is the staple grain.
    - Peanut oil is the main cooking fat.
    - Sushi and any raw fish are carefully prepared.
- **Greek**: Meals are simple but family oriented, with bread being the center of the meal.
    - Cheese, especially feta, is used liberally in the Greek diet.
    - Lamb is favorite meat.
    - Eggs are main dish but not used for breakfast.
    - Vegetables are used as main entrees.
    - Salad with cheese, olive oil, and vinegar are consumed in the Greek diet.
    - Rice is main grain.
    - Rich pastries, like baklava, are used for special occasions.
- **Native American**: Food preferences vary with each region/tribe.
    - Corn, cornmeal, blue corn breads are typical.
    - Corn is a status food for most tribes.
    - Fried foods are common.

- Lard and shortening are main cooking fats.
- **Moslem**: Dietary laws are based on Islamic teachings.
  - Most meats are permitted, except for pork.
  - The Moslem diet prohibits fermented fruits and vegetables.
  - Beans, bulgur, rice are used in many ways as a protein source.
  - Representative foods include bulgur and falafel.
- **Indian**: Many of the health-related problems are related to poverty and inadequate sanitation within the country.
  - Many Hindu people do not eat beef because of the belief in the cow as sacred.
  - Milk is not provided to children in some areas because they believe that milk will hinder growth.
  - Bananas are not given because of the belief that they cause convulsions.
  - Many areas of the country are impoverished, so the food supply may be scant, limited in variety, and deficient of many nutrients.
  - The water supply may not be sanitary. Contamination with pathogenic organisms can cause serious health risk to the people dependent on that water supply. Infant formula prepared with the unsafe water can lead to illness and death in the infant. The nurse may promote breastfeeding because it is more hygienic; designed to perfectly meet human nutritional needs; offers immunologic benefit; is readily available; and not costly to the family.
  - Inadequate sewage handling; insect and rodent infestation; contaminated water; rotting garbage and lack of other waste removal; and presence of disease cause poor sanitation.

Critical Thinking Exercise: Individual and Community

Situation: A client seeks assistance for weight control because she is "tired of being fat". Upon assessment, objective findings include a 46-year-old female, 5′ 5″ tall, and 240 pounds. She also reports feeling out of control with her eating behavior and being disgusted with her physical appearance. The following questions relate to this client:

1. What are two of her major nursing diagnoses?

2. In counseling this client, what are at least three characteristics of dietary principles that should be followed?

3. What diseases might she be at risk for developing as a result of her obesity?

4. For each of the foods in the following list, match them with the culture they are traditionally associated with:

Food	Culture
_____ Bagel	A. Japanese
_____ Baklava	B. Greek
_____ Sushi	C. Native American
_____ Bulgur	D. Jewish
_____ Blue corn bread	E. Moslem

5. Devise a sample menu based on the Food Pyramid for a healthy adult female with an average weight. Develop the dietary plan based on approximately 1800 kcal/day and comprising of 50% of kcal from carbohydrate, 20% from protein, and 30% from fat sources.

Meal	Food	Serving
Breakfast		
Lunch		
Afternoon Snack		
Dinner		
Evening Snack		

Food-Borne Illness

> ### Key Points
>
> • The severity of food-borne illnesses varies with the organism, the susceptibility of the person, and the amount of bacteria or toxin ingested.
> • Control of food-borne disease focuses on strict sanitation and rigid personal hygiene.
> • Home refrigeration temperature is 40 degrees Fahrenheit or lower.

Basic Food Safety Tips

The nurse plays a primary role in nutritional counseling and food safety for persons in all practice settings. Specific interventions to include in dietary teaching include:

• Cook food thoroughly when first cooked.
• Food temperature should be either colder than 40°F or hotter than 140°F.
• If you cook ahead, cool food rapidly in small, shallow containers for storage.
• Food preparation areas must be clean.
• Clean all utensils, dishes, and countertops before preparing food.
• Use hot, soapy water with disinfectant for cleaning.
• Use separate cutting boards for meat and vegetables.
• All persons handling food must follow strict hand washing.
• Wash all fruits and vegetable thoroughly before eating.

Botulism

• Botulism is caused by Clostridium botulinum found throughout the environment.
• Bacteria produce toxin only in a low-acid, anaerobic environment, such as in canned food (vegetables, cured and smoked fish).
• Honey and corn syrup may carry spores.
• The signs and symptoms occur 1-3 days after eating contaminated food, dizziness, weakness, double vision, hoarseness, thirst; death may occur from paralysis of the diaphragm. Botulism mimics flu and appendicitis. The organism can also cause gastroenteritis in children.
• Instruct persons with symptoms to seek medical help immediately because botulism can be fatal.

- Toxins are unstable to heat. Boil home-canned, low acid foods for at least 10 minutes. When home canning, use directions provided by USDA for the use of pressure-cooking.
- Use proper handling for canning and low-acid foods.
- Avoid commercial cans that are bent, bulging, or broken.
- Discard food if a particular odor is noticeable.

Escherichia coli (E. coli)

- Sources are raw ground beef, possibly chicken, and imported soft cheeses due to unsanitary handling of food and unsanitary equipment.
- Signs and symptoms differ with each strain of the *E. coli* bacteria, but may include bloody diarrhea, cramps, fever, chills, dehydration, and kidney problems.
- Sanitary food handling is important.
- Cook ground beef to well-done stage.
- Do not eat undercooked meat or poultry with any red or pink color.
- Avoid cross-contamination between meat and other foods via cooking and preparation equipment/surfaces.

Salmonella

- Sources are found in eggs, poultry, raw milk, and from cross-contamination.
- Signs and symptoms occur 12-24 hours after ingestion and include nausea, vomiting, cramps, diarrhea, chills, and fever.
- Salmonella can be fatal in infants, the elderly, and those with an immunocompromised condition.
- Safe food handling practices are essential, including thorough cooking of all food. Avoid all cross-contamination.
- Prompt and proper refrigeration of foods is necessary to prevent disease.

Shigella

- Shigella is transmitted via fecal-oral routes and less often in contaminated food and water.
- Onset of nausea, vomiting, headache, abdominal cramps, diarrhea, and fever usually occurs after 8-48 hours.
- Shigellosis can be fatal in infants, the elderly, and immunocompromised persons.
- For illness prevention, the nurse educates persons about the importance of thorough hand washing and sanitary food handling and storage.

Campylobacter

- This type of bacteria is found primarily in poultry and somewhat in beef and lamb. Milk can become contaminated with the *Campylobacter jejuni* organism.

- Onset of symptoms of food-borne illness related to *Campylobacter* generally occurs 2-10 days, or longer, after eating.
- Diarrhea, abdominal cramping, fever, and bloody stools may last for 2-7 days.
- The nurse provides nutritional teaching about the importance of thorough cooking of foods, particularly poultry, and sanitization of cooking surfaces in contact with poultry juices.
- Avoid unpasteurized milk.

Listeria

- This type of bacteria, found in soft cheeses made with unpasteurized milk, causes food- borne illness 7-30 days after exposure.
- Physical findings are typically fever, headache, and vomiting, although this infection may be fatal.
- Exposure to listeria during pregnancy can result in fetal loss or birth anomaly.
- Dietary counseling includes information about thorough cooking of foods, sanitary food- handling practices, and avoidance of unpasteurized milk.

Staphylococcus

- Toxin is produced when food contaminated by *staphylococcus aureus* is left for extended periods of time at room temperature.
- *Staphylococcus aureus* is normal skin flora easily transmitted to foods such as potato and pasta salads, cream fillings, pies, milk, poultry, ham, and salad-based sandwich fillings.
- Signs and symptoms occur 2-6 hours after ingestion and include nausea, vomiting, diarrhea, cramps, chills, and fever. This food-borne infection is rarely fatal.
- Refrigerate foods to decrease possibility of organism's growth.
- Toxin is not destroyed by heat, so cooking or boiling does not make the food safe to eat.

Critical Thinking Exercise: Food-Borne Illness

1. Compare and contrast the food-borne illness caused by *Escherichia coli* with that caused by *staphylococcus aureus*.

Food-borne Illness:	Staphylococcus Aureus	Escherichia Coli
Cause		
Signs and Symptoms		
Prevention		

2. Although various governmental agencies are responsible for food safety for consumers, we must also implement our own personal food safety plan. List at least four ways to ensure personal food safety.

Digestion, Absorption, Metabolism, and Excretion

Key Points

1   **Digestion** is the process by which food is broken down in the gastrointestinal tract.

2   **Absorption** is the process by which nutrients are carried into the body's circulation system and delivered to cells.

3   **Metabolism** is the sum of the products of chemical changes in the cell.

4   **Excretion** is the elimination of waste by-products of food breakdown.

Overview

Food that we eat must be changed into simpler substances before our bodies can use them. In the alimentary tract, a series of mechanical and chemical changes occur to reduce food into nutrient compounds needed for health maintenance and growth.

Mechanical Digestion: Process of physically breaking down food into smaller pieces.

- Begins in the mouth with mastication, which is the tearing and grinding effort of teeth and tongue on the food.

- Peristalsis, rhythmic contractions of muscles, helps move food through the gastrointestinal tract.

- Segmentation the forward and backward muscular action, assists in controlling the food mass.

Chemical Digestion: Process of splitting complex molecules into simpler ones.

- Hormones are essential to the digestive process. Gastrin signals the stomach to produce gastric secretions for the protection of the mucosal lining. Secretin stimulates the release of bile by the liver and bicarbonate by the pancreas to aid in digestion. Cholecystokinin causes the contraction of the gallbladder for fat digestion as well as other pancreatic enzymes for protein and carbohydrate breakdown.

- Enzymes are proteins, specific in kind and quantity, that break down specific nutrients. Peptidase is secreted to break down proteins into amino acids. Pancreatic lipase digests fat molecules into essential fatty acid compounds and glycerol. Maltase, sucrase, and lactase aid in the reduction of sugars into fructose, glucose, and galactose. Deficiencies of enzymes can result in poor absorption of protein, fat, or carbohydrate substances.

- Hydrochloric acid and buffer ions produce the correct pH level for digestion.

- Mucous lubricates and protects the mucosal tissues lining the gastrointestinal tract.
- Water transports the products of digestion for absorption and excretion.
- Bile emulsifies fats into droplets.
- Chyme is the mixture of partially digested food with digestive secretions found in the stomach and small intestine.

Absorption

Absorption is the process that carries nutrients into the blood or lymphatic circulation and delivers them to the cells.

- Specialized structures ensure maximum absorption of essential nutrients primarily in the small intestine. The many mucosal folds and finger-like projects of the villi and microvilli increase the surface area of the gut and aid in absorption of nutrients.
- Absorption processes include **diffusion** and **pinocytosis**.

Metabolism

Encompasses the total chemical changes in the body by which it maintains itself. The two fundamental processes are:

- **Catabolism**: Breaking down of food components into smaller molecular particles (destructive phase)
- **Anabolism**: Process of synthesis from which substances are formed (constructive phase)

Excretion

The elimination of unabsorbed materials of digestion in the large intestine.

- Chyme leaves the stomach and passes through the small intestine. Food passes through the ileocecal valve into the cecum and remaining parts of the colon to the rectum until the waste products are eliminated in the feces.
- By-products of digestion normally include cellular wastes, water, bile salts, mucous, undigested food and dietary fiber, and bacteria.

Critical Thinking Exercise: Digestion, Absorption, Metabolism, and Excretion

1. Devise a chart that lists the three major nutrients. Detail the digestive process, beginning in the mouth.

Carbohydrates	
Mouth	
Stomach	
Small Intestine (pancreas)	
Intestine	

Protein	
Mouth	
Stomach	
Small Intestine (pancreas)	
Intestine	

Fats	
Mouth	
Stomach	
Pancreas	
Intestine	
Liver and Gallbladder	

Carbohydrates

Key Points

- All carbohydrates are organic compounds composed of carbon, hydrogen, and oxygen.
- When linked together, simple sugars may form monosaccharides, disaccharides, and polysaccharides.
- Carbohydrates provide energy and fiber.
- Glycogen is the stored carbohydrate energy source found in the liver and muscles.
- Carbohydrate foods generally are widely available, easily grown, and can be stored for long periods of time.
- The ability to digest large amounts of lactose diminishes with age and in persons of various ethnic groups. Lactose intolerance occurring in childhood is related to insufficient lactase production.
- Many carbohydrates are metabolized by bacteria on the teeth and converted to acid resulting in dental enamel erosion and formation of caries.
- Although many fad diets are popular, a balanced diet with reduced sugar is still the most effective way to lose weight and keep it off.

Overview

The main function of carbohydrates (CHO) is to provide energy for the body. CHOs also serve special functions in many other body parts such as the liver and heart. The minimum intake of carbohydrates is 50-100 grams per day. To achieve optimal health, it is recommended that 55-60% of total daily calories come from carbohydrate sources.

Functions of Carbohydrates

- Carbohydrates provide a primary energy resource for the body, breaking down polysaccharides (starches, dietary fiber) into disaccharides (sucrose lactose, maltase) then into monosaccharides (e.g., glucose fructose, galactose).
- Glycogen serves as a vital backup energy source in the liver and muscle tissue.
- Carbohydrates help regulate protein and fat metabolism.
- Carbohydrates help promote normal heart function.
- Carbohydrates are essential for proper functioning of the central nervous system.

Types of Carbohydrates

- Monosaccharides
    - Glucose – corn syrup
    - Fructose – fruits, honey
    - Galactose – milk sugar
- Disaccharides
    - Sucrose (glucose plus fructose) – table sugar, cane sugar
    - Maltose (glucose plus glucose) – sweeteners
    - Lactose (glucose plus galactose) – milk sugar
- Starches
    - Complex carbohydrates contain multiple glucose units chemically bonded together.
    - Glycogen is the storage form of starch in the liver and muscles.
- Dietary fiber
    - The indigestible form of large carbohydrates is dietary fiber.
    - It provides bulk to the stool and aids in elimination of dietary waste.
    - Types of dietary fiber include: pectin, gum, cellulose, and mucilages.
    - Research indicates that healthy amounts of dietary fiber may be likely to reduce the incidence of colon cancer, obesity, and cardiovascular disease.

Digestion

- **Carbohydrates** are digested more quickly and completely than proteins or fats, except for fiber.
- **Cellulose** and some other fibers are non-digestible. Their function is to provide bulk in stool that promotes bowel elimination. There is evidence that cellulose lowers cholesterol.
- **Lactose intolerance** develops in persons with insufficient amounts of lactase. Undigested lactose causes abdominal gas pain and diarrhea.

Absorption

- Absorption occurs mainly in the small intestine using pancreatic and intestinal enzymes.
- The body absorbs 80-95% of carbohydrates.

Metabolism

- **Maintenance** of blood glucose homeostasis at a level of 70-120 mg/dL
- **Glycogenesis**: Process of converting glucose to glycogen
- **Glycogenolysis**: Conversion of glycogen back to glucose
- **Gluconeogenesis**: Producing glucose from fat and protein

Nutritional Counseling

- The nurse should recommend a diet that is high in complex carbohydrates, rather than simple sugars or fat. Starches from whole grains and pasta, cereals, breads, legumes, and beans are necessary for healthy living.
- Carbohydrate intake should be at least 50-100 grams/day and comprise approximately 60% of the total energy intake daily.
- The current advice for sugar intake is moderation, especially between meals.
- Avoidance of high sugar foods accompanied by daily toothbrushing and dental flossing is necessary for the prevention of dental caries and gingivitis.

Critical Thinking Exercise: Carbohydrates

1. List the three categories of carbohydrates, common names for the appropriate ones, and examples of how they occur in natural food sources.

Fats

Key Points

- Fats are a storage form of concentrated energy for the body.
- The chemical group of fats is called **lipids**.
- No more than 20-30% of the total caloric intake should come from fats.
- If the fat content exceeds 30% of total calories, the nurse should emphasize the need for a diet higher in **monounsaturated fat**.
- **Unsaturated fats** come from plant food sources and help reduce health risks.
- **Essential fatty acids**, including omega-3 and omega-6, are important for blood clotting, blood pressure, and inflammatory responses. Omega-3 fatty acids, found in fish, soybean oil, flax seed, and canola can reduce the risk of cardiovascular disease. The Nutritional Committee of the American Heart Association recommends at least two servings of fish per week, especially salmon, for this reason.
- A diet high in saturated fat is linked to cardiovascular disease.
- Saturated fat intake, particularly in dairy products, meats, and greasy or fried foods, should be limited to less than 10% of the total caloric intake.
- Diabetics and persons with pre-existing cardiovascular disease should limit dietary intake of cholesterol and saturated fat to less than 7% of total calories.
- Trans-fatty acid, found in baked goods, fried foods, margarine, and many restaurant foods, containing hydrogenated fat, raise low-density lipoproteins cholesterol. The American Heart Association recommends limiting the intake of foods containing this type of dietary fat.
- Replacing animal protein with soy products can help to reduce LDL cholesterol and triglyceride levels. Cardioprotective effects of soy are indicated for persons with high LDL who are thus at risk for cardiovascular disease. The U.S. Food and Drug Administration allows manufacturers to promote the healthy benefits of foods containing more than 6.25 grams of soy protein per serving.
- Dietary fiber may help to reduce LDL cholesterol levels.

Functions of Fats

- Source of energy
- Palatability of food by adding flavor and texture to foods
- Use as an emulsifier and allow fat and water to mix
- Slows down digestion and makes us feel full and satisfied

- Supplies the essential fatty acids, especially linoleic acid
- Aids in the absorption of fat-soluble vitamins

Types of Fats

Triglycerides: Chemical name for fat. This fatty acid combined with glycerol is necessary to supply energy to the body, allow efficient energy storage, insulate and protect the body, and transport fat-soluble vitamins.

Phospholipids are a class of lipid that is derived from triglycerides. They are important for cell membrane structure.

Cholesterol is another class of lipids, called sterols. Cholesterol is necessary to cell membrane stability and the production of certain hormones and bile salts for digestion.

Saturated fatty acid: Most are solid fats of animal origin

Unsaturated fatty acid: Liquid oil that is usually of plant origin

Essential fatty acid: Linolenic, linoleic, and arachidonic–must be supplied by the diet

Polyunsaturated fat: Of vegetable origin such as corn oil, safflower, and sunflower oil

Digestion of Fats

- Mouth: Small amount of lingual lipase is secretion for initial breakdown of fat.
- Stomach: Small amount of gastric lipase is secreted to cause mechanical separation of fats into smaller components for digestion.
- Fat in the duodenum stimulates the gallbladder to release bile-containing cholecystokinin, which breaks down fat globules.
- Small intestine: Pancreatic lipase further breaks up triglycerides into fatty acids and glycerol.
- Fats are carried to the bloodstream by chylomicron and various lipoproteins, including very-low-density lipoproteins (VLDL), low-density lipoproteins (LDL), and high-density lipoproteins (HDL).

Absorption

- Some fatty acids are absorbed quickly by the villi of the small intestine and then transported directly back to the liver.
- Other longer chains of fatty acids are absorbed later in the terminal ileum.
- Approximately 95% of consumed fat is absorbed, mostly in the duodenum and jejunum.
- Low bile output, high fiber intake, and rapid gastrointestinal motility decrease fat absorption.
- Three factors related to decreased fat absorption are rapid gastrointestinal motility, high fiber intake, and low bile output.
- Steatorrhea is fat in the stool caused by lipid malabsorption. Clients with celiac disease have an inability to digest long-chain fatty acids and an inhibition of pancreatic lipase.

- Addition of medium-chain triglyceride (MCT) oil may be needed to help clients with fat absorption to meet the essential fatty acid requirements for bodily function.

Metabolism

- After entering the bloodstream, lipids are carried to the liver or adipose tissue.
- Lipid metabolism is regulated by lipase.

Major Food Sources of Fat in the United States

- Added fats, oils (shortening, butter, lard)
- Dark meat
- Dairy foods
- Poultry, especially with skin
- Hydrogenated fats in convenience foods

Critical Thinking Exercise: Fats

1. Devise a simple plan for assisting a middle-aged male with high cholesterol and a family history of cardiovascular disease in gradually reducing his saturated fat and cholesterol food intake.

Protein

Key Points

- **Amino acids**, the building blocks of protein, contain usable forms of nitrogen for human life.
- We typically consume more protein than what is needed.
- Undernutrition can lead to protein malnourishment in the form of kwashiorkor or marasmus.
- Protein balance is essential to health and can be used to synthesize glucose when needed.
- It is recommended that 15% of dietary intake come from protein sources.
- Protein requirements are influenced by growth needs and the nature of the diet; adults usually require 40-65 grams/day.
- Of the 20 known amino acids, 9 are essential in the diet because the body cannot manufacture them: histidine, isoleucine, leucine, lysine, methionine, phenylalanine, tryptophan, valine, and threonine. The body synthesizes the rest.
- **Complete proteins** are high quality and contain ample amounts of all nine essential amino acids. Foods containing protein from an animal source provide high biological forms of amino acid.
- **Incomplete proteins** are lower quality and lack sufficient quantities of one or more essential amino acids. Vegetable sources alone lack certain amino acids. A diet containing a variety of plant foods will provide the essential amino acids for growth and health maintenance.
- **Complementary proteins** are two or more food sources combined to compensate for deficiencies in essential amino acid composition in the individual food. Together they yield a high-quality protein. An example of a complementary protein diet the nurse may offer a vegetarian is red beans and rice, green beans and almonds, corn tortillas and beans.
- An **omnivore** is a person who consumes both plant and animal food sources.
- A **vegan** eats only plant foods.
- High-protein, low-carbohydrate fad diets for weight loss can cause serious health problems, including renal dysfunction.

Functions of Proteins

- Primary tissue building
- Growth and maintenance of tissue
- Body's defense system: Lymphocytes and antibodies

- Fluid regulation
- Nitrogen balance
- Transportation of nutrients and other vital substances
- Energy source when carbohydrates and fat are unavailable

Digestion of Protein

- Mouth: Mechanical digestion occurs in the mouth through mastication and excretion of saliva.
- Stomach: Pepsinogen and HCl break protein into smaller polypeptides.
- Small intestine: Polypeptides-pancreatic and intestinal lipase-dipeptides-amino acids are released in the small intestine.
- Pancreas: Trypsin-chymotrypsin and carboxypeptidase-peptides-aminopeptidase and dipeptidase-amino acids are released for digestion of protein.

Nitrogen Balance

- The body's nitrogen balance indicates how well the tissues are being maintained.
- At different life stages and during times of malnutrition and illness, the nitrogen balance may change.
- Positive nitrogen balance occurs when the body takes in more nitrogen than it excretes. It occurs naturally during rapid growth.
- Negative nitrogen balance occurs when the body takes in less nitrogen than is excreted. It may occur with illness and/or malnutrition.

Protein Deficiency Disorders

- **Kwashiorkor** is a protein deficiency disorder that can occur when a child is weaned from human milk and fed high carbohydrate, protein-deficient food. This muscle-wasting disorder can occur as a result of infection or disease.
- **Marasmus** results primarily from extreme starvation. Famine conditions causing a poor intake of protein and energy sources can be fatal, particularly to children. Persons with digestive disorders can also suffer from this type of malnutrition.

Excess Protein Intake

- Research indicates that long-term, high-protein diets can lead to cancer of the colon or elevated homocysteine production.
- Nurses may caution persons with renal dysfunction to avoid a high-protein diet.

Food Sources

- Complete proteins contain all ten of the essential amino acids, usually foods of animal origin (e.g., eggs, milk, meat, and cheese).
- Incomplete protein lacks one or more of the ten essential amino acids, usually foods of plant origin (e.g., grains, legumes, nuts, vegetables, fruits).

Vegetarian Diets

- **Vegan**: eats only plant food.

- **Lactovegetarian**: eats only plant and dairy products.

- **Lacto-ovo-vegetarian**: consumes plant, dairy products, eggs, fish, and occasional poultry.

- An adapted food pyramid for lacto-ovo-vegetarians consists of fruits, vegetables, whole grains, and legumes at the base. The middle tier includes nuts and seeds, dairy products, soy products, egg whites, and plant oils. The top of the pyramid includes eggs and sweets.

- The nurse needs to educate the vegan about the importance of eating good sources of riboflavin, vitamins D and B-12, calcium, iron, and zinc.

- Web sites containing further information:
  - **http://www.oldwayspt.org**
  - **http://www.ivu.org**

Critical Thinking Exercise: Protein

Situation: An 18-year-old healthy female asks you about adopting the vegan style of eating. She is concerned about the health risks of eating meat, and also has strong beliefs about animal rights. Explain some of the benefits of a vegan diet, as well as some of the potential concerns.

1. Benefits of a vegan diet:

2. Concerns related to a vegan diet:

Vitamins

Key Points

- Vitamins are essential organic molecules needed for cellular metabolism, clotting, extrinsic factors, utilization of calcium, and prevention of neural tube defects.
- Deficiency occurs when the vitamin is not consumed in sufficient amounts to meet physiological needs.
- Toxicity of vitamins rarely occurs naturally from food consumption.
- Vitamin supplementation needs are individual and specific.
- Our body needs thirteen vitamins, and each has a specific function.

General Functions

- Control agents in cell metabolism
- Act as components of body-tissue construction
- Prevent specific nutritional deficiency diseases

Vitamins are usually classified as either water-soluble or fat-soluble. Water-soluble vitamins are absorbed in the small intestine and pass into the bloodstream for circulation. Fat-soluble vitamins are considered more stable and resistant to the environmental effects of sunlight, heat, oxidation, and hydration. Deficiencies occur gradually because of the body's ability to store them, particularly in the liver or adipose tissue. This classification of vitamin requires bile for absorption to occur.

Selected Water-Soluble Vitamins and Functions

Water-soluble vitamins are unused by the body and are usually excreted.

- **Thiamine (B1):** Serves as a coenzyme in energy metabolism and in nerve functioning. Deficiency may cause beriberi. Symptoms are evidenced in the digestive tract and occur as anorexia, indigestion, and constipation. Without sufficient quantity of thiamine, the myelin sheaths covering the nerves eventually degenerate, resulting in paralysis and muscle degeneration. Severe deficiency can result in cardiac failure and death. Food sources include lean pork, whole grains, legumes, seeds, and nuts. Antagonists to thiamine are found in raw fish and tea.
- **Niacin (B3):** Involved as a cofactor with many enzymes, especially those involved in energy metabolism. It is the most environmentally stable of the water-soluble vitamins. Deficiency may cause pellagra, which is characterized by the 3 Ds: dermatitis, diarrhea, and dementia. Food sources include protein-containing foods, enriched whole grains, peas, and nuts. Coffee is another rich source of niacin. It may help to prevent pellagra in countries with low-protein food sources.

- **Folate:** Required for synthesis of amino acids and prevention of neural tube effects. Folate, also known as folic acid, is necessary for the formation of DNA and, thus, is important for cellular reproduction in all cell growth and renewal, but especially in the gut, blood, and fetal tissue. Deficiency may cause megaloblastic anemia, impaired cell division, and abnormal protein synthesis. During pregnancy, neural tube defects, such as myelomeningocele or anencephaly, can occur. Pregnant women are advised to consume a diet rich in folate and/or supplemental forms of the vitamin. Early symptoms of folate deficiency are evidenced as swollen gums and a smooth, red tongue. Heartburn, diarrhea, and fatigue also occur with the deficiency state. Alcohol and oral contraceptives can interfere with the absorption of folate. Aspirin, too, has a displacement effect that limits its function. Food sources include green leafy vegetables, citrus fruits, kidney beans, beets, ready-to-eat cereals, and fortified bread. Liver is an excellent source of folate. Because the nutrient value is easily lost in the presence of light and heat, raw vegetables or those cooked for a brief time contain higher functional levels of folate.

- **Ascorbic acid (Vitamin C):** An antioxidant, which aids in tissue rebuilding, and is included in many metabolic reactions. It contributes to wound and fracture healing and is necessary for the formation of collagen for connective tissue formation. Vitamin C is an antioxidant and is more susceptible to destruction by oxygen than either vitamins A or E. This vitamin is important for the adrenal glands to produce adrenaline. Emotional or physical stress increases the body's need for vitamin C nearly fourfold. Iron absorption is facilitated by vitamin C. It acts to enhance the bioavailability of the ferrous compound in the gut. Additionally, vitamin C converts folic acid to an active form, which is necessary for the formation of blood cells and neural tube development in the fetus. Immunologic benefits are reported with high doses although a rebound scurvy phenomenon occurs with abrupt cessation of megadoses. Scurvy is caused by vitamin C deficiency, marked by bleeding problems, and skeletal changes. Some food sources are citrus fruits, sweet peppers, green leafy vegetables, tomatoes, and strawberries.

- **Riboflavin:** Required for growth and vigor; coenzyme in protein and energy metabolism. Deficiency results in cracks at the corners of the mouth and inflammation of the mucous membranes of the mouth and lips (cheilosis), and skin eruptions. Dietary sources include milk, meats, enriched cereals, and green leafy vegetables.

Fat-Soluble Vitamins

- **Vitamin A (retinol):** Needed for vision, tissue strength, and growth. Deficiency may cause night blindness, change in all epithelial tissue, especially oral and vaginal mucosa, or xerophthalmia (abnormal thickening or drying of the eye.) Food sources include fish liver oils, liver, egg yolks, butter, and cream. A large amount of vitamin A in the American diet comes from carotene, which is found in carrots, apricots, sweet potatoes, squash, and cantaloupe.

- **Vitamin D (cholecalciferol):** Needed for its antioxidant action, which prevents cellular structures from being broken down by oxygen-free radicals. Vitamin D acts more like a hormone in the utilization of calcium. Deficiency results in rickets, osteomalacia, hemolytic anemia, and damage to nerve fibers that affect walking and vision. Food sources include vegetable oils, cod liver oil, fortified milk, and eggs. Sunlight is another major source of vitamin D in the skin.

- **Vitamin E (tocopherol):** Needed for its antioxidant action, which prevents cellular structures from being broken down by oxygen. It is stored in adipose tissue. Vitamin E is stable to heat and acidic pH but easily destroyed by light, oxygen, and alkaline pH. This vitamin will maintain its integrity with normal cooking temperatures, but not frying. Deficiency results in hemolytic anemia and the nerve fibers that affect walking and vision. Very large supplemental doses of 60 times the RDA for a year or longer may result in toxicity symptoms including bleeding, impaired wound healing, and mental depression. Food sources include vegetable oils, milk, and eggs.

- **Vitamin K:** Functions primarily in blood clotting. Deficiency may result in blood clotting problems. Over consumption of foods high in vitamins A and E may interfere with the liver's use of vitamin K. The body is capable of synthesizing some vitamin K in the large intestine by intestinal bacteria. Food sources include liver, milk, green leafy vegetables, and vegetables in the cabbage family. The typical American diet supplies approximately 5-10 times the RDA requirements for average, healthy adults and children.

- **Toxicity:** Excess intake of fat-soluble vitamins may lead to toxicity because they are not readily excreted and can accumulate in the body, in the liver, and adipose tissue. Toxicities of vitamins A and D are the most common. Vitamin E and water-soluble vitamins C, B6, and niacin can also cause toxic effects, but only when consumed in very large amounts (15- 100 times the normal human need).

- **Absorption** of fat-soluble vitamins depends on the body's ability to absorb dietary fat. Fat digestion is mediated by bile salts and the enzyme lipase and depends on the integrity of the small intestine. Cystic fibrosis, celiac disease, Crohn's disease, and other diseases involving impaired fat absorption will lead to poor utilization of fat-soluble vitamins. Medications, such as the weight-loss drug orlistat (Xenical), can interfere with fat absorption and, therefore, impair the ability to use fat-soluble vitamins.

Critical Thinking Exercise: Vitamins

1. For each of the following vitamins, state the major function and a food source:

- Thiamine (B$_1$)

- Niacin (B$_3$)

- Folate

- Vitamin A (retinol)

- Vitamin K

2. Where are water-soluble and fat-soluble vitamins absorbed?

3. Pellagra is a niacin deficiency disorder characterized by specific symptoms. Which physical manifestation can occur with pellagra?

Minerals

Key Points

- Major minerals are essential and are required daily in amounts of 100 mg or more.
- Trace minerals are required daily in amounts of <20 mg.
- Mixed diets of a variety of foods are the best sources of minerals.
- The nurse should advise persons to follow a diet plan such as the Food Guide Pyramid that offers a wide variety of foods. The use of fortified foods or vitamin supplements may provide the necessary vitamin and minerals for health promotion and illness prevention.

Overview

The seven major minerals are calcium, phosphorus, sodium, potassium, magnesium, chloride, and sulfur. Prime sources for minerals include both plant and animal foods. Minerals are usually considered very stable when cooked. There are eighteen trace elements, which are also essential, but occur in trace amounts in the body.

Selected Major Minerals and Functions

- **Calcium:** Functions in bone and tooth formation, blood clotting, muscle and nerve action, and metabolic reactions. It is best absorbed in the presence of vitamin D. Calcium deficiency may result in tetany or osteoporosis. Physical assessment signs are Trousseau's sign and Chvostek's sign. Food sources include milk and dairy products, grains, egg yolks, and green leafy vegetables. Lactose deficiency causes gastrointestinal symptoms if dairy products are consumed. Calcium-fortified foods and juices and calcium supplements may be needed to meet the RDA of 800-1200 mg/day. Weight-bearing activity can help promote bone remodeling. Calcium toxicity is reported only in cases of excessive intake of calcium supplements.
- **Potassium:** Functions in water balance, metabolic reactions, muscle action, insulin release, and blood pressure. Deficiency may be a result of diuretic therapy and may affect cardiac function. Other symptoms of hypokalemia include muscular cramping, loss of appetite, constipation, and confusion. Food sources include unprocessed foods, oranges, tomatoes, prunes, avocados, cantaloupe, bananas, milk, and broccoli. The minimum daily requirement for potassium is 2 gm/day. Average adequate intake is 2-3.5 mg/day. Potassium toxicity occurs when kidney function is compromised. Hyperkalemia can result in potentially fatal cardiac dysrhythmias.

- **Sodium**: Helps regulate fluid balance, conducts nerve impulses, allows muscular contractions, and many metabolic reactions. Sodium depletion can occur with excess perspiration, persistent vomiting, and diarrhea. This state results in muscular cramping, nausea, vomiting, shock, or coma. The absolute minimum sodium requirement is 100 mg/ day for survival. The American Heart Association recommendation for sodium intake is 2400 mg/day. The typical American diet contains 4-7 gm/day.

- **Phosphorus**: Functions in bone and tooth formation, energy transfer of DNA and RNA, a buffer in formation of phosphoric acid, and balancing acid-base levels. Deficiency of phosphorus is unknown. It is widely available in all foods, especially protein-rich foods and cereal grains. It is also found in convenience foods and soft drinks. RDA is 800-1200 mg/day. Phosphorus deficiency can occur in premature infants receiving long-term parental fluid, alcoholics, elderly persons with nutrient-poor diets, vegetarians, persons with long-standing diarrhea, and high doses of aluminum-containing antacids. A balance of phosphorus with calcium is important in preventing phosphorous toxicity; under- consumption of calcium in the diet can lead to excess phosphorous in the system.

- **Magnesium**: Most is found in our bones and is important for structure and storage. It acts as a catalyst for many enzyme reactions in the body, which affect nerve and muscle function, including the actions of the heart, and also has a role in blood clotting. Deficiency tends to be from secondary causes such as excessive vomiting and diarrhea. Food sources include whole grains, legumes, broccoli, and leafy green vegetables. Milk, meat, and grains contain a sufficient amount of magnesium for bodily function. Hard water also contains high magnesium content. Refined food is a poor source of magnesium. RDA is 280-350 mg/day.

- **Chloride**: Assists in maintaining fluid balance and is a component of hydrochloric acid. Deficiency is rare as adequate amounts are easy to consume. Dietary sources include table salt and what is naturally found in many foods. RDA is 750 mg/day.

- **Sulfur**: A component of protein and vitamin structures. Sulfur functions in acid-base balance. There is a deficiency only if protein-malnourished, and is found in all protein- containing foods. RDA has not been established to date.

- **Fluoride**: Forms a bond with calcium, which means that fluoride accumulates in calcified body tissues such as bones and teeth. Fluoride's main function is to prevent dental cavities.

Selected Minor Minerals and Functions

- **Iron**: Responsible for hemoglobin function, cellular oxidation of glucose, antibody production and synthesis of collagen. Food sources include liver, organ meats, egg yolks, and whole grains, as well as dark green vegetables. Vitamin C increases the absorption of iron.

Critical Thinking Exercise: Minerals

1. Our bodies absorb calcium based on physiological need. Which factors tend to impact calcium absorption? Address factors such as high fiber diets, lactose, dietary fat, and sedentary lifestyle.

Water

Key Points

- Adult water consumption should be approximately 8-10 cups/day.
- **Fluid homeostasis** is essential for optimum health and bodily function. The balance of fluid and electrolytes is a dynamic process regulated by the hypothalamus in the production and release of hormones, including **antidiuretic hormone** (ADH) and **aldosterone**.
- **Intracellular fluid** is water inside the cells.
- **Extracellular fluid** is made up of the water between the cells (**interstitial fluid**) and inside the bloodstream and lymphatic system (**intravascular fluid**).
- **Osmolarity** is the concentration of active particles in a solution.
- **Osmolality** is the number of dissolved particles per volume of fluid.
- **Edema** is the excessive accumulation of interstitial fluid that is often seen in persons with congestive heart failure, renal disease, severe protein deficiency, hypothyroidism, and pregnancy-induced hypertension.

Overview

A typical adult has 55-65% of his total body weight as water. The water composition is greater in muscular tissue than fat. Water intake recommendations for adults are 1.0-1.5 mL of water for each calorie expended under normal conditions, which equals approximately 2 liters per day. Typical urinary output is 1.5-2.0 liters per day. Other sources of fluid loss are in the forms of stool, tears, and insensible water loss through evaporation, perspiration, fever, vomiting, wounds, or infection. The average person can survive approximately 8 weeks without food, but only a few days without water. Primary sources of water should be water instead of soft drinks, alcohol, coffee, and tea.

Functions of Water

- Helps to regulate body temperature through the process of **evaporation**
- Acts as a lubricant in joints
- Cushions body tissues
- Transports nutrients and waste products
- Participates in chemical reactions
- Acts as a solvent and enables minerals and other chemicals to undergo biological reactions in the body

Fluid Compartments

- **Intracellular fluid** is all fluid contained within the cell. The majority of the body is comprised of intracellular fluid. Water passes through the cell membranes in and out of the cell to maintain fluid balance and meet bodily needs.
- **Extracellular fluid** is all the fluid outside the cell. This type of bodily fluid is lost more rapidly outside of the cell itself. The total body weight is made up of approximately 20% extracellular fluid. Components of extracellular fluid are:
  - **Interstitial fluid**: the fluid between and surrounding the cells
  - **Intravascular fluid**: the fluid within the blood vessels
  - **Lymph fluid**: the fluid circulating within the lymphatic system
  - **Transcellular fluid**: fluids in the bodily compartments of the synovial joints, spinal column, intraocular cavities, tympanic structures, intestinal tract, and pericardial and pleural compartments

Fluid Transport

- **Osmosis** is the movement of body water across a semi-permeable membrane to normalize the concentration of particles on each side of the membrane.
- **Diffusion** is the movement of body water or ions to an area of high concentration of particles to an area of lower concentration of particles.

Bodily Fluid Regulation

Physiologic mechanisms controlling the balance of water and electrolytes primarily involve the release of various hormones and the renal system. The hypothalamus helps the body to regulate water balance through the thirst mechanism and release of antidiuretic hormone (ADH) and aldosterone. ADH is released from the pituitary gland when the blood is too concentrated. It signals to the kidney to hold on to water for dilution. Aldosterone is the hormone secreted by the adrenal glands causing retention of sodium ions for a concentration effect. The kidneys respond to ADH and aldosterone release by producing other enzymes that regulate water and electrolyte retention or excretion.

Clinical Water Balance

Water loss can be due to environmental (temperature, physical activity), functional (vomiting, diarrhea), or metabolic (demands of body function) factors.

Dehydration

- Contributing factors to fluid volume deficit:
  - Diarrhea, vomiting, high fever, sweating, diuretics, polyuria, strenuous physical exercise, inadequate intake, or excess ADH (such as diabetes insipidus)
  - Quicker dehydration among elderly persons and infants
  - Assessment findings: decreased skin turgor, confusion, weakness, low urine output, concentrated urine, sticky (dry) mucous membranes
- Dehydration may occur for some of the same reasons as fluid volume deficit.

Warning signs include pronounced thirst, loss of coordination, dry skin, mental confusion, and decreased urinary output. Thirst should not be used as an accurate gauge for fluid needs since it is not triggered until dehydration has already begun.

Overhydration

- Contributing factors to fluid volume excess:
  - Sodium retention, excessive IV fluids, water intoxication (psychiatric condition), too little ADH (such as in syndrome of inappropriate antidiuretic hormone), side effect to medication (such as corticosteroids)
  - Assessment findings: edema, hypertension, crackles in lungs, heart murmur, third heart sound, cough, and shortness of breath
- Overhydration may occur for the same reasons as fluid volume excess. A serious form of overhydration is called water intoxication and occurs when a person consumes large volumes of water within a short period of time. It can cause muscle cramps, decreased blood pressure, and weakness. There may be a psychological component to this disorder.

Special Liquid Diets

- **Clear liquid** diet includes the intake of transparent fluid often served at room temperature. Typical selections are gelatins, tea, broth, white grape juice, soft drinks, and popsicles. A clear liquid diet may be ordered for clients undergoing various diagnostic procedures. Usually in the post-anesthesia period, clients require a clear liquid diet until the intestinal tract returns to normal function. Those experiencing nausea, vomiting, and diarrhea may require this type of diet to rest the gut until normal peristalsis returns. Although the clear liquid diet provides a source of hydration to maintain fluid homeostasis, longer-term needs for protein, fat, and other nutrients are not provided. Cautious use is warranted for use of this dietary restriction for greater than 48 hours. Attention is warranted for clients with hypertension, renal disease, Ménière's disease, and other health conditions because the clear liquid diet often contains high caffeine and sodium solute loads.
- **Full liquid** diet typically includes milk, custard and pudding, ice cream and sherbet, thinned hot cereal, soup, fruit smoothies, and breakfast drink. As a client's diet is advanced from NPO status through the introduction of liquids to solids, the liberalized diet helps the gut to gradually tolerate and digest more.

Critical Thinking Exercise: Water

1. The body's requirement for water varies according to several factors. List and explain at least three of these factors.

Pregnancy

Key Points

- **Energy** needs are increased during pregnancy for the development of the fetus and supporting organs, such as the placenta. Approximately 300 kcal/day are needed to meet the added metabolic demand for fetal growth.
- **Maternal nutritional demands** are increased for development of the placenta, enlargement of the uterus, formation of amniotic fluid, increase in blood volume, and preparation of the breast for lactation.
- **Protein** requirements are also increased to support the growth and development of fetal tissue. An additional 10 grams/day is considered minimum to maintain health fetal and maternal changes during pregnancy.
- Increased **vitamin** needs, particularly for folate and vitamin C, are necessary for the formation of blood, absorption of iron, and development of fetal tissue, such as connective tissue and neural tube structures. Excessive Vitamin A consumption during pregnancy can cause birth defects. This is a result of the liver storing large amounts of Vitamin A, and toxicity resulting.
- **Mineral** requirements, including iron, are more important during pregnancy because of its use for oxygen transport in the blood.

Overview

Diet and health habits prior to and during pregnancy will influence the health status of the mother and baby. The goal of prenatal nutritional education is to prepare the woman for the physiologic changes and to aid her in meeting the demands of pregnancy on her body and the growth and development of the fetus. The Special Supplementation Food Program for Women, Infants, and Children (WIC) provides nutritious food to low-income women who are pregnant or lactating, and their children under age 5. Food vouchers are available for milk, eggs, cheese, juices, fortified cereals, and infant formula.

Nutritional Needs

- **Energy**
  - Increased energy intake of approximately 300 kcal/day is needed to accommodate the rise in maternal basal metabolic rate (BMR), as well as to support the development of maternal and fetal tissues.
  - Breast tissue develops in preparation for lactation, thus, requiring added energy supply.

- Uterine growth and formation of amniotic fluid increase the metabolic demand during pregnancy.
- Energy needs are even higher during pregnancy in the adolescent woman, whose body demands for growth are already increased.
- **Protein**
  - The RDA for protein during pregnancy is 60 grams/day to support the rapid tissue growth for maternal and fetal structures.
  - Amniotic fluid is made of albumin, which is a form of protein.
  - Developing blood volume requires added dietary protein during pregnancy.
- **Vitamins**
  - **Folate** (vitamin B_3) is necessary for the prevention of neural tube defects and megaloblastic anemia. Daily intake of 400-600 mcg/day is recommended in the dietary or supplemental form.
  - **Vitamin C** is important for the conversion of folate to an active form, the absorption of iron in the digestive tract, and formation of connective tissue in the fetus.
  - **Vitamin B** complex, including thiamine, riboflavin, and niacin, has many functions for maternal and fetal metabolism.
- **Minerals**
  - **Iron** is needed for the manufacture of hemoglobin in the maternal and fetal red blood cells. Iron needs double during pregnancy and usually require supplementation to achieve the RDA of 30 mg/day. Iron deficiency is common during pregnancy because of the great demand. Close monitoring of hemoglobin and hematocrit during pregnancy is important for the prevention of this complication. Dietary sources of iron may include dried beans, dates, figs, prunes, and whole wheat.
  - **Calcium** requirements rise during pregnancy because of bone mineralization in the fetus. The RDA for calcium at this time is 1200 mg/day. Calcium is also important for lactation. Milk products offer a rich calcium source that is highly available for absorption.
  - **Iodine** plays a role in the formation of the thyroid hormone. During the second half of pregnancy, the woman's need for iodine increases by approximately 25%.
  - **Fluoride** is important for the development of teeth in the fetus. Dental structures begin in the first trimester of gestation. Supplemental fluoride of 1 mg/day is effective in strengthening teeth and the prevention of caries later in life.
- **Water**
  - The pregnant woman is advised to drink 6-8 ounce servings of water per day.
  - Dehydration is linked to premature labor, maternal urinary tract infection, and various antenatal complications.

Nutrition Related Concerns

- **Caffeine** intake during pregnancy should be limited to promote rest in the mother. Some studies indicate an association of high caffeine intake with low birthweight in the infants. Abrupt withdrawal of high caffeine supply at birth can result in apnea in the newborn.

- **Tobacco** use during pregnancy is linked to prematurity, placenta previa, abruption placenta, and low birthweight. Some studies report an association between maternal smoking and increased risk of sudden infant death syndrome (SIDS).

- **Weight gain** during pregnancy is normally 2-4 pounds/week in the first trimester, then generally 1 pound/week after that. Total weight gain in the woman with healthy pre- pregnancy baseline weight is recommended to be 25-35 pounds and somewhat less in the obese woman. Insufficient weight gain can result in intrauterine fetal growth impairment.

- Hormone changes cause normal **morning sickness**. Eating small, frequent meals and snacks, taking in fresh fruits and vegetables, avoiding high-fat foods, and serving foods cold or at room temperature instead of hot, can relieve nausea associated with pregnancy. Hyperemesis gravidarum is a potentially serious complication that can result in dehydration and poor nutritional status for mother and fetus.

- **Heartburn** is common during pregnancy due to the hormonal effect on the sphincter above the stomach. The enlarging uterus often causes upward displacement of the diaphragm, which tends to increase symptoms of gastric reflux. It can be minimized by a diet low in fat, avoidance of recumbent position after meals, and elimination of spicy foods, alcohol, and tobacco from the diet.

- **Constipation** is common during pregnancy because of the slowing of peristalsis and increasing uterine pressure on the intestines. A high-fiber diet, including at least 30 gm/ day, is particularly important at this time. Generous fluid intake can also help to lesson symptoms of constipation.

- **Leg cramps** may be related to insufficient calcium or excess phosphorous. Calcium supplements with increased intake of milk or other dietary sources of calcium are recommended to prevent this type of neuromuscular irritability.

Critical Thinking Exercise: Pregnancy

Situation: A 35-year-old primigravida is in her seventh month of pregnancy. Her total weight gain so far has been six pounds. Prior to becoming pregnant, she was approximately 40 pounds above ideal body weight. She is concerned about gaining too much weight during her pregnancy.

1. What nutritional information should you provide her?

Lactation

Key Points

- A breastfeeding mother continues to provide all of her baby's nutritional needs.
- Milk production requires energy, about 800 kcal/day.
- Some of the energy needs are met by fat stored during pregnancy, so only an additional 500 kcal/day is needed via the diet.
- Protein needs increase during lactation by 15% for a total of 65 g/day.

Overview

The number of mothers choosing to breastfeed has increased and currently 2/3 of white women and 1/4 of black women breastfeed. Well-nourished mothers who breastfeed exclusively provide adequate nutrition from birth to 15 months. Solid foods are introduced at about 6 months of age. Hormones (Prolactin, Oxytocin) released in response to the suckling infant promote secretion of colostrum and then milk production in 2-3 days.

Benefits of Breastfeeding to the Mother

- Convenience and economy
- Promotes mother-infant bonding
- Facilitates uterine contractions and controls postpartum bleeding
- Promotes return to pre-pregnancy weight
- Decreases the risk of ovarian and premenopausal breast cancer

The basic diet followed during pregnancy should be continued during lactation Other considerations are to continue prenatal vitamin supplements, increase fluids, and to have the proper amount of rest and relaxation.

Energy and Nutrient Needs

- Increase calories to 500-800 per day, depending on the volume of milk production.
- Increase protein by 15% for a total of 65 g/day.
- Avoid certain foods only if they create a problem for the infant (e.g., cabbage, onions)
- Adequate fluid intake is essential. Fluid should be replaced through drinking water, milk, or juice. Coffee and cola should be avoided, as the caffeine acts as a

stimulant and its effects are passed on to the infant. Alcohol should be avoided as it inhibits oxytocin; thus, it inhibits the letdown reflex.

Contraindications to Breastfeeding

- Pre-existing maternal diseases such as breast cancer, AIDS, active tuberculosis, malaria, herpes simplex, lesions of breast, and chicken pox in the first three weeks post partum
- Maternal alcoholism and/or drug addiction
- Maternal mental illness

Critical Thinking Exercise: Lactation

1. Discuss the two hormones for lactation. Include the "let-down" reflex and inhibitors of that reflex.

Infant Nutrition

Key Points

- Term infants need approximately 110 kcal/kg/day during first 6 months of life and then 100 kcal/kg/day from 6 months to first birthday.
- Preterm infant energy requirements are 120-150 kcal/kg/day or greater, depending on gestational age and metabolic needs.
- Infant birth weight doubles in 4-6 months and triples by the end of the first year of life.
- Breast milk or iron-fortified formula provide the essential nutrients to support normal growth in infancy.
- Protein requirements are highest during the first 4 months of life.
- Infant fetal stores of iron are depleted at about 4-6 months after birth. Supplementation or iron-fortified cereal is necessary at that time.
- **Failure to thrive**, defined as inadequate gains of weight and height during infancy, may be related to physical illness, poor maternal-infant bonding, lack of physical touch, and emotional negligence.
- Common feeding concerns in the first year include: colic, constipation, diarrhea, milk intolerance, and iron-deficiency anemia.

Overview

In the first year of life, the weight of an infant is expected to triple, with a 50% increase in length. In order to support this rapid growth and development, there must be adequate energy provided. The role of the health professional in caring for infants is close monitoring of the growth patterns for weight, length/height, and head circumference. Growth charts may be accessed at the National Center for Health Statistics web site at http://www.cdc.gov/nchs.

If a mother decides not to breastfeed, there are a variety of commercially-prepared formulas available. The infant's primary care provider should determine which formulashould be used. These formulas are available as either "ready-to-feed", or as a powder or liquid concentrate. Cow's milk is not advisable for children under one year old because of the risk of iron-deficiency anemia.

Benefits of Breastfeeding for Baby

- Boosts the immune system for protection against infection and disease
- Safe from bacterial contamination
- Lessens the risk for ear infections
- May enhance development of the nervous system

- Contributes to maturation of the gastrointestinal system
- More easily digested
- Less diaper dermatitis
- Reduces risk of food allergies
- Likely to enhance maternal-infant attachment
- Establishes a habit of eating in moderation

Breastfeeding Guidelines

- Breastfeed infant for 6 months or longer, if possible. Then introduce infant formula when breastfeeding declines or ceases.
- The infant sucking stimulus sends a nerve impulse to the mother's hypothalamus to secrete prolactin, and also to initiate the release of oxytocin. The more often the infant nurses, the more breast milk will be produced. To increase the supply of milk, offer the breast or pump more often.
- The breast should be offered 10-12 times per 24 hours in the first several weeks. Nursing each breast for 10-15 minutes is a good guideline.
- Milk is produced by supply and demand; the more the baby nurses, the more milk is produced.
- Offer no bottles of formula or water while milk supply is being established.
- Iron levels deplete at age 4-6 months; therefore, supplementation of iron should be established at 1mg/kg/day.
- Do not thaw frozen breast milk in the microwave because it destroys immunologic properties and may have hot spots, resulting in burn to infant's mouth.
- Provide iron-fortified cereal at 4-6 months of age.
- Feed a wide variety of soft foods after 6 months of age.
- Investigate the need for fluoride supplementation if the water supply is not fluoridated.
- Investigate the need for iron supplementation if the infant is preterm or at risk for iron- deficiency anemia.

Breastfeeding Preterm Infants and Multiples

- As multifetal pregnancy is often preterm, infants would benefit even more from the protection offered by breast milk.
- Delay in offering the breast to the preterm infant may be necessary until after 33-34 weeks gestation, if medical condition is stable. Prior to this time, the suck-swallow reflex is immature and the infant is at increased risk for aspiration, tiring, and expending excess calories needed for growth. Pumped breast milk may be offered by intermittent or continuous enteral feeding routes, depending on the status of the baby.
- Breastfeeding multiples allows time for attachment and emphasizes the bonding process.
- Twins may be fed both at once or separately. Feeding them together cuts down

on the amount of nursing time; this is especially beneficial during the night.

- Diet and fluid needs of the mother are particularly important during lactation for multiples. Encourage high protein snacks and up to 80 ounces of fluid per day.
- Investigate the need for iron supplementation for preterm infants.

Formula-Fed Infant Nutrition Guidelines

- Term infants generally require 32 ounces/day of formula during the first few months of life.
- Complete and written instructions should be given to parents on how to prepare the formula.
- Stress the importance of mixing formula exactly as written on the label.
- Use cold tap water for preparation, allowing water to run for two minutes to reduce the chance of lead in the formula.
- Never heat formula in a microwave because of the possibility of hot spots.
- Discard unused formula after two hours.
- Formula should be iron-fortified to prevent anemia.
- Add iron-fortified cereal to the diet at 4-6 months of age.
- Provide a variety of soft foods after 6 months of age as tolerated.
- Never prop bottles because of the risks of choking, as well as dental caries later in infancy. Holding the infant is crucial for maternal-infant bonding.

Solid Food Guidelines and Feeding During the First Year

Solid foods may be added at around 4-6 months of age, after the infant's gastrointestinal system has matured. Earlier introduction may result in increased allergies and gastrointestinal upsets.

- Be sure the infant is developmentally ready to take solid food. That means the infant is able to sit with support, can move jaw, and protrusion reflex is gone.
- After 6 months of age, introduce one food at a time with a 5-day interval between new foods.
- Begin with iron-fortified infant cereal and follow with strained fruits or vegetables.
- Do not add salt or sugar to the diet.
- Avoid the introduction of egg whites and chocolate prior to 1 year of age to prevent the development of food allergy.
- Avoid feeding the infant the following foods during the first year: hot dogs, hard candy, raw carrots, popcorn, nuts, and peanut butter to prevent the possibility of choking.
- Do not give a baby honey or corn syrup because of the risk of botulism.
- Cow's milk in the infant less than a year of age may lead to iron-deficiency anemia. After 1 year, offer whole or 2% milk to provide the essential fatty acids needed for optimum brain development.
- Failure to thrive may occur due to organic causes such as congenital heart

disease or non-organic causes when there is no medical reason for poor growth. Psychosocial causes may include poor bonding, poverty, child abuse, or neglect.

- Avoid excessive amounts of apple or pear juice. The high fructose content can cause diarrhea. Fruit juice that is offered instead of formula can cause deficiencies in calcium and other minerals necessary for growth and development of bone and tissue. Studies have also shown the link of high juice intake to obesity and poor dental health.

Common Feeding Concerns in the First Year

- **Colic** is presumed abdominal discomfort occurring in healthy infants. Repeated crying episodes lasting 3 hours or longer that do not respond to normal soothing remedies is considered colic. It affects approximately 10-25% of babies. Typical crying episodes occur in late afternoon or early evening. In the absence of other physical symptoms, the crying baby flexes legs into the abdomen, clenches fists, or responds with rigid posture. The breastfeeding mother is advised to continue nursing the baby, but should reduce caffeine and nicotine-containing products, which can aggravate the condition. Restriction of maternal diet for foods including beans, broccoli, onions, or garlic is controversial.

- **Milk intolerance** occurs in less than 5% of infants receiving formula. The rare occurrence in the breastfed infant may be corrected with elimination of milk products in the mother. Symptoms usually include diarrhea, vomiting, abdominal distention, and blood in the stool. One-quarter to one-half of the infants treated with a soy-based formula will achieve only temporary relief of symptoms and may eventually develop an allergy to soy. Predigested formulas may be needed for true milk intolerance.

- **Iron-deficiency** anemia typically occurs in older infants who are weaning and not receiving an iron-rich diet. This nutritional deficiency occurs when the infant receives excessive cow's milk. Supplemental iron may be necessary.

- **Diarrhea and constipation** are common concerns, particularly to the first-time parent. Breastfed infants rarely become constipated. Normal breast milk stools are looser in form than that of the formula-fed infant and may be passed with every feeding. True diarrhea in the infant can lead to dehydration. Intravenous fluid replacement may be necessary to prevent potentially fatal complications.

Critical Thinking Exercise: Infant Nutrition

Situation: Parents of a 6-month-old infant want to know more about introducing solid foods to their child's diet.

1. What instruction might you give them?

2. What nutritional information should be given to a mother who is breastfeeding twins or multiples?

Childhood Nutrition

Key Points

- The increased growth rate of infancy slows down by about the age of 1 year.
- Growth occurs unevenly until puberty.
- Children model eating behaviors of adults.
- Nutrition guidelines should be modified as needed but still ensure RDAs.
- The rapid growth during infancy tapers during the preschool years. The appetite of the preschool child also diminishes when the metabolic need decreases.
- A diet low in saturated fat can provide adequate nutrients for growth and development. It is important to eat foods that are dense in nutrients and low in calories.

Overview　　　As children grow, their eating habits change. Caregivers are the best nutrition educators for their children. Dietary Guidelines for Americans are appropriate for children in regard to the 30% or less fat intake and the emphasis on fruits, vegetables, and complex carbohydrates.

Guidelines for Toddlers

- Mealtime consistency is important.
- This is a good time to start the "One Bite Rule" as a way to expose the child to a wide variety of acceptable food sources.
- Mealtime atmosphere should be relaxed and conducive to conversation.
- Allow children to self-feed as much as possible.
- Energy requirements are about 1300 Kcal/day.
- Protein needs increase to 16 g/day.
- General guideline for portion of food is one tablespoon per year of age. The toddler's stomach holds about one cup at a time.
- Introduce a variety of foods.
- Provide whole milk or formula until age 2 years and then switch to low-fat or skimmed.
- Finger foods are easy for the toddler to eat. At this age, they also begin to break, tear, snap, and dip food. They are able to start using a spoon, especially if hungry.

- Toddlers are typically picky and sporadic eaters. Food preferences are frequently marked by "food jags."
- Many toddlers have the tendency to put food in their mouths and hold it there without swallowing.
- Children who are receiving oral iron supplements should have orange juice added to the diet to increase the absorption of iron.

Guidelines for Preschoolers

- The stage of 4-6 years (preschool) is characterized by independent eating styles.
- The 6-year-old child should weigh twice as much as he/she did 1 year prior.
- Snacks are essential, and should be nutritious. Encourage introduction of new foods, including fresh fruits and vegetables, whole grain breads and cereal, milk, and other nutrient-dense foods. Encourage the child to at least taste new foods.
- Children at this age typically master developmental tasks involving autonomy. They respond better to food choices, rather than demands. They can participate in selecting some healthy foods or snacks. Preschoolers tend to have strong likes and dislikes and may protest to the point of tears. An awareness of smells, appearance, and texture influences their opinions. Familiar foods are generally accepted better than new ones.
- Energy requirements are up to 1800 kcal/day, and protein increased to 24 g/day.
- The average height gain is usually 3-4 inches (7.5-10 cm) and weight gain is 4.5-6.5 pounds (2-3 kg) during this time.
- Avoid mealtime struggles. Although guiding the child to eating healthy foods often requires tenacity and perseverance, the commitment to teaching the child to like healthy foods will benefit for a lifetime.
- Dexterity is improving. The preschool child is now able to use a spoon and fork, and cut with a dull knife. He/she can pour milk and juice into a cup and serve an individual portion from a larger bowl. The average child of this age is capable of peeling, spreading, cutting, and mashing foods. Cracking an egg or peeling a carrot is enjoyable for most preschoolers.

Guidelines for School-Age Children

The school-age child, 7-12 years, is characterized by slow growth as the body is preparing for the puberty growth spurt. The Food Guide Pyramid for children ages 2 through 6 is available at http://www.usda.gov/cnpp.

- Body types are established and growth rates vary widely.
- A good breakfast is very important for learning to occur.
- School lunch programs provide a nourishing meal.
- Peer influence at school lunchtime increases.
- Energy requirements increase to 2000-2200 kcal/day and protein increases to 28-46 g/ day depending on sexual maturity.
- Obese children are more likely to become obese adults. It is particularly important to teach this child to select healthy food choices and engage in regular, vigorous exercise. With early intervention, the patterns that can lead to this health risk can be thwarted as the child continues to grow in height.

- Increased bone growth requires increased calcium from 800 mg/day at age 10 to 1200 mg/day through adolescence.
- Healthy snack choices may include fruit, yogurt, and low-fat cheese.

Health-Related Nutritional Concerns

Baryophobia

- **Baryophobia** is a condition in which children are underfed because of the caregiver's fear of future obesity or cardiovascular disease later in life.
- Social desirability for thinness influences the caregiver to provide the same low-fat, low-calorie diet that adults consume for weight management. However, the food choices may be insufficient to meet the nutritional needs of a growing child, resulting in a pattern of poor weight gain.
- The child suspected to have baryphobia should be monitored closely for patterns of weight gain and height increase.

Critical Thinking Exercise: Childhood Nutrition

1. Age-appropriate, nutritious snacks are important during childhood. List some healthy and attractive alternatives to refined sugar for a 9-year-old.

Nutrition During Adolescence

Key Points

- The final growth period during childhood occurs at the time of puberty.
- The rate of growth varies widely and is dependent on genetics, nutrition, and hormonal influences.
- Initially, the boys' growth spurt is slower than the girls', but boys soon catch up and exceed girls.
- Eating patterns are influenced by rapid growth and peer influences.
- During the adolescent growth period, the physiologic need for calcium and iron increase. The bone matrix laid during these years can establish or prevent the risk for later development of osteoporosis in adulthood.

Overview

Females need about 2200 kcal/day and 45 g/protein/day. Males need 2500-2900 kcal/day, and 45-59 g/protein/day. Calcium recommendations for both genders are 1200 mg/day. Energy requirements are higher than at any other period in life.

Overall Diet Plan

The recommended overall diet plan for adolescents should be balanced and contain a variety of vegetables, fruits, whole grains, and higher-protein foods. Many teens are concerned about weight and appearance, often trying to reach unhealthy weight for height and frame. Peer pressure and media influences for thinness may affect the adolescent's self-image and perceived appearance. Studies have revealed that only one-quarter of teenage girls who consider their weight to be normal are still actively dieting for weight loss. The extreme diet or fad diet to achieve unhealthy weight can have far-reaching, physiologic effects on hormones for female reproduction and menstruation, bone modeling, gastrointestinal disease, and eating disorders.

Nutritional Problem Concerning Calcium

Calcium is of special concern to allow for skeletal growth and bone mineralization. Milk remains a primary and excellent source of calcium, and teenagers should be encouraged to drink it daily. If drinking milk is avoided, it may be useful to include it in cereals or soups. carbonated drinks in place of milk can lead to inadequate calcium intake. Additionally, Carbonated drinks contain a high level of phosphorous, which leeches calcium from the bones and can increase the risk for fractures. A snack of yogurt and cheese is also an option for meeting physiologic needs for dietary calcium. Other dietary sources of calcium include fortified fruit juices, the cheese on pizza, sunflower or sesame seeds, and raisins.

Snacking

- Nourishing snack foods should be readily available.
- Fast foods typically contain increased calories, fats, and decreased vitamins A and C.
- It is important to include breakfast and lunch in daily meal pattern.

Lactose Intolerance

- Lactose intolerance is caused by a deficiency of lactase and occurs in almost 50% of the population worldwide.
- Undigested lactose causes abdominal cramping, flatulence, and diarrhea.
- Commercially prepared lactose-free products are now available. These products also contain increased amounts of calcium.

Iron-Deficiency

- Adequate iron intake is important for males whose rapid growth makes it necessary to increase blood volume and lean body mass.
- Adequate iron intake is important to females particularly after the onset of menses.
- Iron-rich foods include beef, liver, pork, lamb, chicken, shellfish, egg yolks, salmon, whole grains, lima beans, green peas, almonds, green leafy vegetables, raisins, apricots, tomatoes, and strawberries.

Anorexia Nervosa

- Eating disorder of self-imposed starvation
- Most common in adolescent females
- Distorted body image results in inability to see themselves as underweight
- Tendency to be overly perfectionistic, introverted, and perhaps socially insecure
- May include binge eating and compulsive behavior, such as extreme exercise
- Physical signs and symptoms include amenorrhea, cardiovascular difficulties, electrolyte imbalances, dehydration, metabolic alkalosis or acidosis, loss of muscular strength, low blood pressure, and lanugo.

Binge-Eating Disorder

- Binge-eating disorder is characterized by recurrent episodes of binging, feeling out of control when eating at least 2 days a week for 6 months or more.
- Consuming more than the average portion in a discrete period of time accompanied by the sense of lack of control during the episode
- Binge episodes usually occur when the person is alone because of the embarrassment of the amount and type of food consumed.
- Purging occurs in response to binging, through use of laxatives and/or self-induced vomiting
- Binge foods are typically high-calorie and high-fat, requiring minimal preparation.

- Obsession with body shape and weight and the binge/purge may be triggered by a stressful event.
- Binge-eating disorder is frequently associated with ineffective coping skills.
- Physical findings include weight fluctuations, fatigue, poor dental health, enamel erosion, dehydration, electrolyte and acid/base imbalances, sore throat, esophageal rupture, and cardiac arrhythmias, and calloused index finger from self-stimulated purging.

Critical Thinking Exercise: Nutrition During Adolescence

1. Anorexia is a psychological disorder characterized by self-imposed starvation. List the psychological and physical manifestations of anorexia.

Psychological	Physical

2. What recommendations would you make to an adolescent who has lactose intolerance in order to maintain an adequate calcium intake?

Nutrition During Adulthood

Key Points

- Life expectancy has increased from 47 years in 1900 to 77 years in 2000.
- Women outlive men by an average of six years.
- Overall physical growth levels off in early adult years.
- Some of the physical changes of aging affect food patterns, preferences, and ability to prepare adequate meals to meet nutritional needs for healthy living.
- Lack of sufficient nourishment is the primary nutritional problem of older adults.
- Herbal and nutritional supplements are not regulated by the federal Food and Drug Act (FDA). Limited research supports therapeutic uses for many of the supplements available commercially. However, caution is warranted because they may be potentially harmful to some. It is generally advisable to use only one product at a time, observing for deleterious effects. Consult with care provider prior to use.

Overview

By the time an individual reaches age 24, growth levels off and the body achieves a state of balance. The basic energy and nutrient needs of an individual adult will vary according to living and working conditions. There is no evidence that healthy adults require additional nutritional supplements if the dietary intake includes wide variety of healthy foods, such as those recommended in the Food Pyramid. Adults should choose whole grains, fruits, and vegetables daily. They should also select foods low in saturated fat and cholesterol and moderate in total fat. Choosing foods with less salt is a practice to aid in regulating body fluids and lower blood pressure. Foods and beverages with low or moderate amounts of sugar will help to control weight and maintain teeth free of caries. The consumption of alcohol should be moderate, as moderation is associated with lessened risk of cardiovascular disease and stroke. Nitrate-containing foods from the meat curing and smoking process may increase the risk of certain cancers and should be avoided.

Early Years (20s & 30s)

- Transition from one stage of lifespan to another
- Young adults who are living independent from families and focusing on personal and career goals are at increased risk for nutritional challenges.
- The childbearing years present demanding nutritional needs for women.

- Females need approximately 2200 kilocalories and 46-50grams/protein per day.
- Males need approximately 2900 kilocalories and 58-63 grams/protein per day.
- Calcium and phosphorus 1200 mg/daily until age 24, then drops to 800 mg/daily
- Dietary patterns established during early childhood usually last a lifetime.

The Middle Years (40s & 50s)

- Increased stress and responsibility of raising children
- Empty nest syndrome
- Family meals no longer a requirement, so may eat out more often
- Regular exercise and positive dietary patterns can delay or prevent non-insulin-dependent diabetes mellitus and coronary artery disease.
- Females after age 50 need 1900 kilocalories/day, but protein requirements stay the same.
- Males need 2300 kilocalories/day; protein requirements remain unchanged.
- Iron requirements for females decrease to 10 mg/day once menstruation ceases.

The Older Years (60s & beyond)

- Level of wellness may reflect health behaviors.
- Retirement may be a delight for some and for others a loss of social status.
- Focus on continued fluid needs by drinking eight 8-oz. cups of water per day.
- Nutrition may be affected by availability of finances, transportation, and living conditions.
- The older adult may need increased vitamins D and B12.
- Physical changes may result in inability to eat and/or constipation.
- With impaired mobility, less social support, altered sensory perception, and reduced appetite; the elderly are at risk for malnourishment. This group may benefit from home- delivered meals, congregate services, and other related community support services to support nutritional health.

Calcium Needs

- In general, calcium needs decrease after age 24 since skeletal growth has finished.
- RDAs drop from 1200 mg/day to 800 mg/day.

Cholesterol Levels

- Cholesterol levels are determined by genetic factors, fat, cholesterol content of the diet, obesity, and activity levels.
- As low-density lipoprotein (LDL) cholesterol levels rise, so does the risk of coronary artery disease.
- Saturated fat, especially in animal and dairy products, is linked to higher LDL cholesterol levels.

- Current guidelines recommend reducing total fat intake to 30% of total kilocalories, <10% saturated fat, and <300 mg cholesterol per day.

- A lower saturated fat diet combined with weight reduction will usually lower LDL cholesterol levels. Replacement of foods high in saturated fat with a diet containing polyunsaturated fat is recommended.

- The Nutritional Committee of the American Heart Association endorses a limitation of 300 mg/day. Persons at risk for cardiovascular disease, those with a history of high LDL cholesterol levels and diabetics should maintain a diet with less than 200 mg/day.

- Studies have shown that consumption of shellfish and eggs does not significantly raise LDL cholesterol levels.

Antioxidants

- Antioxidants are compounds that guard other compounds from oxidation.

- Vitamins C and E work together as antioxidants to destroy substances released as cells age or become damaged.

- Vitamin E and beta-carotene may prevent oxidation of fats, thereby helping to prevent heart disease. Dietary sources are more bioavailable than vitamin supplements.

- Vitamin C may limit the development of atherosclerotic plaque in the arteries.

Critical Thinking Exercise: Nutrition During Adulthood

1. The elderly person may be at increased risk for dehydration. Causes may range from senility and simply forgetting to drink, to consciously limiting fluids to avoid increased urination at night. List the common signs and symptoms of dehydration.

2. State some of the risk factors that may be associated with malnutrition in the elderly.

Food, Nutrient, and Drug Interactions

Key Points

- All medications have the potential for side effects and risks.
- The amount and rate of medication absorption can be affected by the composition and timing of food intake.
- A proper diet can reduce the risk of altered effectiveness of some medications.

Overview

Determination of risk for nutrient-medication reactions depends on individual assessments including: age, physiological status, multiple medication intake, liver and kidney function, and normal dietary patterns.

Effects of Medications on Food

- Oral medications must first be broken down and dissolved in gastric juices before they can be absorbed.
- The rate of medication absorption may increase or decrease, based on the amount and quality of food in the stomach.
- Appetite stimulant medications include:
    - Antidepressants, such as amitriptyline (Elavil)
    - Antihistamines (Claritin), such as cyproheptadine hydrochloride (Periactin)
    - Steroids, such as hydrocortisone
    - Tranquilizers, such as lithium and diazepam (Valium)
- Appetite depressant medications include:
    - Amphetamines, such as Dexatrim and Dimetapp
    - Antiarrhythmics, toxic levels of digoxin (Lanoxin)
    - Antibiotics, such as metronidazole hydrochloride (Flagyl)
- Antidepressants, such as fluoxetine hydrochloride (Prozac)
- Other medications may react by altering taste, including:
    - The antiarrhythmic drug doxazosin mesylate (Cardura)
    - Antihypertensives, such as captopril (Capoten)
    - Anticonvulsants, such as phenytoin (Dilantin)
    - Anti-gout medication, such as allopurinol (Zyloprim)

- Medication absorption is enhanced when taking the following medications:
  - Acetylsalicylic acid (aspirin)
  - Propoxyphene hydrochloride (Darvon)
  - Propranolol hydrochloride (Inderal)
  - Nitrofurantoin sodium (Macrodantin)
  - Metoprolol tartrate (Lopressor)
  - Spironolactone (Aldactone)
  - Hydralazine hydrochloride (Apresoline)
- Medication absorption is diminished upon taking the following medications:
  - Amoxicillin (Amoxil)
  - Penicillin G (Wycillin)
  - Tetracycline (Achromycin)
  - Phenytoin (Dilantin)
  - Astemizole (Hismanal)
  - Dipyridamole (Persantine)
  - Phenobarbital sodium (Luminal)

Effects of Medications on Nutritional Status

- Medications can alter food intake, nutrient absorption, metabolism, and excretion.
- Anticoagulants may interact with vitamins C, E, K by either increasing or decreasing bleeding time.
- Anticonvulsants may interact with folic acid or vitamin D and decrease calcium absorption.
- Antipsychotics interact with vitamin B2 to cause a mild deficiency.
- Cephalosporins interact with vitamin K to cause deficiency.
- Hypokalemia causes digoxin toxicity.
- Antibiotics may disrupt folate metabolism.
- Excretion of nutrients may be altered by poor drug excretion.
- Diuretics may result in a potassium deficiency.
- Monoamine oxidase (MAO) inhibitors have been reported to cause hypertensive crisis when used with tyramine-rich foods. Foods to avoid include cheeses, wines, beer, smoked or dried fish, and yeast products.

Effects of Alcohol on Nutritional Status

- Alcoholism is a primary cause of vitamin and nutritional deficiencies.
- Nutritional problems occur because the person substitutes alcohol for food, and because alcohol is toxic to body cells.
- The under-consumption of nutritious food leads to insufficient amounts of thiamine, niacin, folic acid, and vitamins A and C to meet bodily needs.
- Chronic alcohol ingestion leads to liver dysfunction. The client develops low serum albumin, resulting in fluid third spacing into body tissues. Clinically, the

- client appears edematous and may have ascites and jaundice.
- Alcohol-related deficiencies might result in loss of muscle strength, bruising, poor healing, bleeding gums, anorexia, diarrhea, social irritability, depression, anxiety, dementia, peripheral neuritis, liver dysfunction, and hypoproteinemia (e.g., albumin).

Effects of Food on Medications

- The types of food consumed may affect medication absorption.
- If absorption is increased by the presence of food, medication should be taken with a meal or snack.
- If medication absorption is decreased by the presence of food, absorption occurs best if medicine is taken 1 hour before or 2 hours after eating.

Critical Thinking Exercise: Food, Nutrient, and Drug Interactions

1. Many medications have unpleasant side effects that are not caused by the illness. The side effects range from mild to severe. A common side effect of medications is gastrointestinal tract irritation and discomfort accompanied by nausea. List some nursing interventions that may be used to alleviate this particular side effect.

Enteral Nutrition

> ## Key Points
>
> - When the gastrointestinal tract is used to provide nourishment, the feeding is referred to as **enteral nutrition**.
> - Therapeutic nutrition is the role of food and nutrition in the treatment of diseases and disorders.
> - As long as possible, regular oral feedings are preferred.
> - A therapeutic diet involves the modification or adaptation of the basic, normal diet, according to the needs of the client.
> - Collaborate with the dietician for nutritional or eating problems.

Overview

The basic diet becomes therapeutic when it is modified in any one of the following ways: calories are increased or decreased, fiber is increased or decreased, specific nutrients are increased or decreased, specific foods are omitted for various reasons, and any modification to make the foods soft or liquid, based on clients' needs.

Clear Liquid Diet

- It consists of foods in the clear and liquid form served at room temperature.
- Clear liquid diet is without residue and is non-stimulating and non-gas forming.
- Inadequate in providing proteins, minerals, vitamins, and kilocalories
- It is important to avoid excess caffeine consumption, which could lead to increased hydrochloric acid (HCl), and stomach upset, as well as sleeplessness
- Indications for a clear liquid diet include acute illness, postoperative recovery, reduction of colon fecal material prior to certain diagnostic tests and procedures.
- A clear liquid diet should not be used for longer than 24 hours, except in cases of inadequate gastrointestinal function.
- Acceptable foods are water, tea, coffee, fat-free broth, carbonated beverages, clear juices, ginger ale, and plain gelatin.
- Clients who are on fluid restrictions may benefit from lemon wedges in beverages, which will stimulate saliva and moisten a dry mouth.

Full Liquid

- Consists of foods that are liquid at room temperature
- Provides oral nourishment for clients having difficulty chewing or swallowing solid foods.
- Full liquid offers more variety and nutritional supplements than a clear liquid diet and can supply adequate amounts of energy and nutrients.
- If used longer than 48 hours, high-protein, high-calorie supplements should be considered.
- Indications include a transition between liquid and soft diets, postoperative recovery, acute gastritis, febrile conditions, and/or intolerance for solid foods.
- Clients with dysphagia need to be cautious with liquids, unless they are thickened appropriately.
- Foods allowed are all liquids on clear liquid diet, all forms of milk, soups, strained fruits and vegetables, eggnog, plain ice cream and sherbet, plain gelatin.

Pureed

- Offer pureed or strained foods or other foods with a smooth consistency to clients having difficulty chewing or swallowing (e.g., fractured jaw, cerebral vascular accident).
- The composition and consistency of a pureed diet varies, depending on the client's needs.
- Each food is pureed separately to preserve flavor.
- Adding small amounts of liquids such as broth, milk, or gravy facilitates appropriate consistency.
- Pureed diets are modified for special dietary needs (e.g., sodium, fat, calorie).

Mechanical Diet

- Texture of food is modified slightly in a mechanical soft diet.
- A mechanical diet includes foods that require minimal chewing before swallowing (e.g., ground meats, canned fruits, soft-cooked vegetables).
- Indications: Poorly-fitting dentures, edentulous, limited chewing or swallowing, dysphagia, or strictures of the intestinal tract
- Modified for other dietary restrictions also

Soft Diet

- A soft diet contains whole foods low in fiber and only lightly seasoned, which are easily digested.
- Food supplements or between-meal snacks are used to add calories.
- Indications: Transition between full liquid and regular diet, acute infections, chewing difficulties, gastrointestinal disorders

Regular Diet

- A regular diet is indicated for clients who do not need dietary restrictions.
- Many health care facilities offer self-select menus for regular diets.
- Dietary modifications to accommodate individual preferences, food habits, and ethnic values can be done without difficulty for the client receiving a regular diet.

Diet as tolerated is ordered to permit client's preferences and situation to be taken into consideration. The nurse may assess the client for hunger, appetite, and nausea when planning the most appropriate diet, after consulting with a dietician.

Critical Thinking Exercise: Enteral Nutrition

1. Plan a sample menu for a client who is on a soft, low-fat diet. Include food selections for breakfast, lunch, and dinner.

Enteral Tube Feeding

> ## Key Points
>
> - Enteral tube feeding is a liquid diet of a formula instilled via a tube inserted into the gastrointestinal tract.
> - Tube feeding requires a functioning gastrointestinal tract.
> - Tube feedings consist of blenderized foods or a commercial formula administered by a tube into the stomach or small intestine.
> - Enteral method most closely utilizes the body's own digestive and metabolic routes.
> - The liver is very important in tube feeding because it extracts, processes, alters, and metabolizes the nutrient.

Overview

Enteral tube feeding is used when the client cannot consume adequate nutrients and kilocalories orally, but still has a functioning gastrointestinal tract.

Feeding Routes

- **Nasogastric tube** is passed from nose to stomach.
- **Nasointestinal tube** goes from nose to jejunum.
- **Gastrostomy tube** endoscopically or surgically inserted into stomach.
- **Jejunostomy tube** surgically inserted into small intestine.
- The anticipated length of time that tube feeding will be required determines the type of tube used.
- Endoscopic or surgical placement is preferred when long-term use is anticipated, or when obstruction makes insertion through the nose impossible.
- Placement into the stomach simulates normal gastrointestinal function.

Tube Feeding Formulas

- Commercial products are preferred over home-blended ingredients because they provide a known nutrient composition, controlled consistency, and bacteriological safety.
- Polymeric formulas are composed of intact nutrients that require a functioning gastrointestinal tract. They provide 1-2 kilocalories/mL and include blenderized foods, milk-based products, high-calorie, and lactose-free products.

- Elemental formulas (predigested) contain 1.0-1.3 kcal/mL and are used for clients with a partially functioning gastrointestinal tract, or those who have impaired capacity to digest foods. They are lactose-free and are not very palatable.
- Modular formulas provide 3.8-4.0 kcal/mL and are not nutritionally complete by themselves.

Tube Feeding Complications

- Most tube feeding complications are preventable.
- Gastrointestinal complications include constipation, diarrhea, cramping, pain, distention, and nausea and vomiting.
- Mechanical complications include tube misplacement, aspiration pneumonia; irritation and leakage at the abdominal tube site; irritation of nose, esophagus, and mucosa, and tube lumen obstruction. Feeding tube obstruction can be prevented with flushing of the tube after use and avoidance of dry products and medications. The use of liquid medications is preferred to prevent blockage of the tube.
- Metabolic complications include dehydration, hyperglycemia, hyper or hyponatremia, and overhydration.
- Gastrostomy tube feedings are well tolerated because the stomach chamber holds and releases feedings in a physiologic manner that promotes more effective digestion. As a result the "dumping syndrome" is usually avoided.

Nursing Considerations

- Nasogastric tubes can migrate; it is essential for nurses to monitor correct placement of tubes by measurement, auscultation, X-rays, and client comfort level.
- Always wash hands before handling formula or enteral products.
- To maintain the patency of the feeding tube, the nurse flushes it routinely with warm water.
- To check for proper placement of the feeding tube, the nurse aspirates residual content. Small-diameter feeding tubes may be difficult to aspirate.
- Hold feeding if residual is greater than 100 mL. Notify the primary care provider.
- Assess and monitor:
  - Airway patency
  - Oxygen saturation
  - Breath sounds
  - Bowel sounds
  - Bowel elimination
- Elevate head of bed to at least 30° during and 30 minutes after feedings to lessen the risk of aspiration.
- Administer feeding solution at room temperature to decrease gastrointestinal discomfort.

- Fill bag with approximately 4 hours worth of formula to minimize bacterial growth in unrefrigerated formula.
- Replace feeding bag and tubing every 24 hours to prevent bacterial growth.
- Begin with a small volume or dilute formula to prevent diarrhea. Increase concentration and volume in intervals until full strength is reached.
- Store unused portion in a refrigerated place in a covered container for up to 24 hours. Label the formula with the name, room number, and date the formula was opened.
- Feeding schedules may include:
  - Continuous
  - Cyclic
  - Intermittent
  - Bolus
- A client who is NPO will require meticulous oral care and comfort measures, such as ice chips.
- Some persons may require nutrition support service at home for long-term enteral nutrition. A multi-disciplinary team, including the nurse, dietician, pharmacist, and primary care provider monitors the weight, electrolyte balance, and overall physical condition of client discharged with this type of nutritional therapy.

Critical Thinking Exercise: Enteral Tube Feeding

1. List and describe some of the nursing considerations for safely administering enteral tube feedings.

2. One of the most common complications of tube feeding is diarrhea. List two possible causes and the treatment for each.

Parenteral Nutrition

Key Points

- Total parenteral nutrition (TPN) is used when a client's gastrointestinal tract is not functioning or when caloric needs are very high.
- TPN solution composed of >10% dextrose can only be administered in a central vein.
- Peripheral parenteral nutrition must be isotonic and contain less than 12.5% dextrose.
- Monitoring, administration, tubing change, and site care varies among institutions. Provide care according to unit protocol.

Overview

Parenteral nutrition may be used when the client is unable to absorb nutrients or needs an increased amount of kilocalories. Other indications include high-dose cancer chemotherapy, radiation, pancreatitis, severe malnutrition, major surgery, malabsorption disorders, inflammatory bowel disease, major trauma, and burns.

Total Parenteral Infusion

- TPN typically includes water, amino acids, dextrose, electrolytes, vitamins, and trace elements and is infused into a peripheral or intravenous site.
- Lipid solution is added either by "piggyback," a secondary infusion every three days, or adding it directly to one bag of the TPN solution.
- Carbohydrate solutions are available in concentrations of 5% through 70%. Healthy adults need 2 grams glucose/kg/day.
- Amino acids: Protein is provided as a mixture of essential and non-essential amino acids.
- Fats: Lipids are used as a concentrated energy source, as well as to prevent essential fatty acid deficiency.
- Electrolytes and minerals are added and are essential for normal body functions and to prevent diseases reflected in deficiencies.
- Vitamins are added according to RDAs.
- Trace elements (zinc, copper, manganese, chromium, and selenium) are added to prevent deficiencies.
- Insulin may be added to reduce potential for hyperglycemia.

Nursing Care

- Nursing care is directed at preventing complications through consistent monitoring.
- Specific monitoring guidelines vary among different healthcare facilities.
- Monitor urine glucose and vital signs every six hours, and monitor serum glucose at least daily.
- Weight, intake and output, and electrolytes (first three days only) are checked daily.
- CBC, electrolyte panel, PT/PTT, BUN, and cholesterol are done as a baseline and then repeated weekly.
- Use sterile technique when changing central line dressing and tubing.
- Change the bag and tubing with sterile technique every 24 hours.
- Prepare solution in a sterile location at the pharmacy and keep refrigerated.
- Electronic infusion device is used to prevent accidental overload of solution.
- Monitor clients for "cracking" of TPN solution. This occurs if the calcium or phosphorus content is high or if low-salt albumin is added. A "cracked" TPN solution has an oily appearance or a layer of fat on top of the solution, and should not be used.

Complications

- **Technical complications** include: pneumothorax, subclavian artery puncture, catheter embolus, air embolus, thrombosis, obstruction, and bolus infusion.
- **Septic complications** include: catheter-related sepsis, and/or thrombosis.
- **Metabolic complications** include: hyperglycemia, hypoglycemia, hyperkalemia, hypophosphatemia, hypocalcemia, and hypoalbuminemia.

Critical Thinking Exercise: Parenteral Nutrition

1. Discuss clinical settings where parenteral nutrition:

- Should be part of routine care:

- Usually would be helpful:

Gastrointestinal Disorders

Key Points

- Diseases of the gastrointestinal tract and its accessory organs interrupt the body's normal cycle of digestion, absorption, metabolism, and elimination.
- Nutritional management of gastrointestinal disease is based on the degree of interference in the normal process of digestion.
- Food intolerances and allergies may manifest as gastrointestinal symptoms.
- Diseases of the accessory organs also contribute to nutritional problems.

Overview

Disorders of the gastrointestinal tract include those affecting the esophagus, stomach, and the small and large intestines. Accessory organs supporting digestion are the gallbladder, pancreas, and liver. Disorders may result in tissue inflammation and pain, lactose intolerance, and dysphagia. Many disorders are influenced by lifestyle choices.

Dysphagia—Difficulty swallowing

- Dysphagia is common after prolonged intubations, major surgery, stroke, and disabling traumas.
- Approximately 35% of nursing home residents have dysphagia.
- Signs and symptoms: unexplained decrease in food intake, repeated pneumonia, very slow chewing, frequent throat clearing, holding pockets of food in the cheeks, drooling, coughing.
- Diets need to be individualized and include thickened foods and adequate fluid volume.
- Safest eating positions are either upright or with HOB elevated and supported with pillows.
- Staff supervision is necessary during mealtime for clients with dysphagia; encourage small bites and chewing thoroughly.

Gastroesophageal Reflux and Hiatal Hernia

- Gastroesophageal reflux disease (GERD), also known as acid reflux, is a burning sensation that occurs in the upper chest from stomach acid backing up into the esophagus. This acid irritates the lining of the esophagus, causing pain.

- Hiatal hernia is a protrusion of a portion of the stomach through the esophageal opening. The symptoms are similar to GERD and are managed likewise. Occasionally, surgical intervention is necessary to relieve the pain.

- Some underlying causes are poor cardiac sphincter muscle tone and hiatal hernia. Pregnancy and obesity are associated with increased production of estrogen and progesterone, which relax lower esophageal sphincter tone, causing reflux of stomach acid. Adipose tissue turns certain circulating hormones into estrogen.

- Constant regurgitation of acid gastric contents into lower part of esophagus causes chronic irritation.

- Signs and symptoms: severe heartburn occurs 30-60 minutes after eating, pain radiates to neck, jaw, or down the arm; vocal changes, pain upon bending over or lying down.

- Management of symptoms:
  - Manage weight within healthy parameters.
  - Avoid lying down until at least 2 hours after meals.
  - Sleep with head of bed (HOB) elevated.
  - Use antacids to neutralize the acid, such as Tums, Gaviscon, and Maalox.
  - Over-the-counter H2 blockers work by reducing the production of acid, such as Tagamet, Zantac, and Pepcid.
  - Proton pump inhibitors are extremely effective in suppressing acid, such as Prilosec and Prevacid.
  - Surgical intervention may be necessary for severe and long-lasting symptoms.
  - Drink plenty of water when taking medication to prevent further irritation of the esophagus.
  - Eat small, frequent meals.
  - Chew foods well.
  - Avoid milk, pepper, caffeine, alcohol, acidic juices, fat, chocolate, and mints.
  - Quit smoking.
  - Avoid tight-fitting clothing.

Peptic Ulcer Disease

- Peptic ulcer disease (PUD) is defined as an open lesion in gastric or duodenal mucosa. Duodenal ulcers are found more commonly in young persons and gastric type in older adults.

- A combination of factors contribute to the development of an ulcer in a susceptible person:
  - Genetic predisposition
  - Smoking
  - Dietary factors, such as calcium, alcohol, and spicy foods
  - Histamine
  - Certain medical conditions

- Nonsteroidal anti-inflammatory drugs (NSAIDs) and aspirin
- *Helicobacter pylori*
- Stress
- The leading cause of peptic ulcer disease is the acid-resistant bacterial infection caused by H. pylori. This bacterial infection has recently been found to be contagious with a long asymptomatic period.
- Tissue damage results from gastric acid and pepsin in the ulcerative process. The primary risk is complete erosion of the stomach lining, causing gastric or intestinal perforation and subsequent peritonitis. Additionally, the ulcer may cause damage to the blood vessel, leading to massive blood loss, shock, and death.
- Tissue damage is also seen secondary to use of NSAIDs and aspirin.
- Other potential causes may be cigarette smoking, genetic predisposition, and stress. It is important to stop exposure to nicotine, and to reduce the stress level as much as possible.
- Incidence peaks in persons aged 50-70 years.
- Clinical signs and symptoms occur as a result of increased gastric muscle tone and painful contractions when stomach is empty.
- Eat nutritious meals with adequate amount of dietary fiber on a regular schedule. Avoid strong spices and acidic foods.
- In the past, foods containing milk and cream were recommended to soothe and protect the stomach lining. Today it is known that these substances increase the acid and mucous production, aggravating ulcer formation, and should be avoided.
- Maintain a healthy weight.
- Treatment includes:
  - Reduction of stress
  - Proper rest
  - Acid-blocking agents
  - Mucosal protectors
  - Antibiotics
  - Antacids
  - Diet therapy
- Avoid large doses of aspirin, ibuprofen, and other NSAID compounds unless otherwise prescribed. Newer NSAID medications that contain prostaglandin reduce gastric acid production and enhance mucous section.
- The basic goal of diet therapy is to support healing and prevent further tissue damage. The nurse encourages a diet that is caffeine-free and bland. Alcohol, tobacco, and milk- based products should be avoided to decrease the excessive secretion of gastric acids. Eat small, frequent meals.

Lactose Intolerance

- Lactose intolerance is a deficiency of any of the disaccharides in the small intestine, primarily lactase.

- The deficiency produces multiple gastrointestinal symptoms, including gas and abdominal pain.

- Lactose intolerance results from insufficient lactase, causing abdominal cramping and diarrhea.

- Milk and milk products need to be avoided.

- Soymilk products and milk treated with a lactase product can be used. Lactrase is a pharmacologic supplement for lactose.

- Restricting milk may result in a calcium, riboflavin, and vitamin D deficiency, and supplementation may be needed.

- Some medications use lactose fillers (e.g., Benadryl, Calan, Dyazide, Inderide-LA, Librax, Librium, Premarin).

Irritable Bowel Disease

- Irritable bowel syndrome (IBS) is most commonly seen in the form of ulcerative colitis or Crohn's disease. Ulcerative colitis is an inflammatory disease of the large intestine that spreads the ascending portions of the bowel. Crohn's disease is also an inflammatory disease affecting localized portions of the bowel. Characteristically, healthy segments alternate with diseased areas. Symptoms of IBS include diarrhea, constipation (alternating), bloating, and abdominal cramping. A feeling of incomplete elimination after a bowel movement is common. Stools contain mucous and are usually loose in consistency.

- May develop because of a genetic predisposition or as a result of long-term, low-fiber eating habits and increased intracolonic pressure, such as straining with stool.

- During periods of inflammation, the goal is to rest the bowel, achieve bowel rest with NPO and progress to clear liquids.

- The nurse recommends the person with IBS to avoid dairy products and gas-producing foods, such as legumes, cauliflower, broccoli, grates, raisins, cherries, and cantaloupe. Popcorn and other seeds and nuts are prohibited.

- Small volume feedings are helpful as large meals trigger contractions to the large intestine.

- Reduction of stress is therapeutic.

- As inflammation resolves, gradually increase fiber content; add gradually to prevent side effects such as flatulence, cramps, and diarrhea.

Critical Thinking Exercise: Gastrointestinal Disorders

1. Discuss a nursing care plan that deals with the responsibility for feeding clients with dysphagia. Include safe procedures and features of foods to be considered.

2. List at least four dietary treatment guidelines for peptic ulcer disease. Include the rationale for each.

Liver, Gallbladder, and Pancreas Disorders

Key Points

- The liver, gallbladder, and pancreas produce important digestive agents that enter the intestine and aid in breaking down food substances.
- Medical nutrition therapy is part of the treatment for disorders of these organs and is necessary to prevent nutritional deficiencies.

Overview

Disorders of the gastrointestinal tract include those affecting the esophagus, stomach, and the small and large intestines. Accessory organs supporting digestion are the gallbladder, pancreas, and liver. Disorders may result in tissue inflammation and pain, lactose intolerance, and dysphagia. Many disorders are influenced by lifestyle choices.

Cirrhosis

- Chronic degenerative disease in which liver cells are replaced by the buildup of fibrous tissue and fatty liver changes.
- Alcohol, hepatitis, metabolic diseases, or chronic use of hematoxic medications may cause the damage.
- Low plasma levels result in low colloidal osmotic pressure. This leads to third spacing and reduced circulating intravascular volume. The client appears edematous and may develop ascites. Diuretic therapy is a treatment for ascites. Monitor potassium levels with loop therapy.
- Diet therapy includes decreased protein initially to 20-40 g/day then increased protein to 80-100 g/day as tolerated to correct malnutrition. Monitor blood ammonia levels to assess client's ability to process protein.
- Sodium is restricted to 500-1000 mg/day to reduce ascites.
- Soft textured food prevents damage and possible rupture of esophageal varices.
- The client with cirrhosis requires increased kilocalories, vitamins, and minerals. It is critical that no alcohol is consumed.
- In liver failure, the dietary protein is restricted to reduce ammonia levels and encephalopathy.

Cholecystitis

- Acute inflammation of the gallbladder is usually associated with gallstones.
- Risk factors for gallbladder disease include increased age, being female, obesity with high fat intake, hormonal imbalances, certain medications such as oral birth control pills and insulin, enzyme deficiencies, and very low-calorie diets for weight loss.
- Signs and symptoms include fat intolerance, flatulence, belching, epigastric heaviness, heartburn, and chronic upper abdominal pain after eating, nausea, and vomiting.
- During an episode of acute cholecystitis, the client is managed with IV fluid therapy and NPO. Chronic cholecystitis is treated with low-fat diet and weight loss, if indicated.
- Surgical removal of gallstones or gallbladder may be needed.

Cystic Fibrosis

- An autosomal, recessive inherited disease of the mucous-producing exocrine glands.
- Occurs one in 2500 live births. One in 20 Caucasians carries the recessive gene.
- Signs and symptoms include increased levels of sodium and chloride in saliva and tears, highly viscous secretions in pancreas, bronchi, bile ducts, and small intestine.
- Nutrition is of prime importance.
- Poor nutritional status (undernutrition) leads to poor growth and pulmonary complications.
- Primary goal of nutritional therapy is to increase kilocalories and all other nutrients, particularly protein.
- For the person with cystic fibrosis, the protein needs are nearly doubled.
- Fat intake can be boosted with supplementation using medium-chain triglyceride solutions.
- A special form of fat-soluble vitamin is necessary because of the dysfunctional exocrine activity to break down fat compounds.
- Pancreatic enzyme, vitamin, and mineral supplements are essential for growth and health maintenance.
- Additional salt is usually needed, especially during hot weather, febrile illness, or physical exertion.
- Zinc deficiency is common because of excess passage in the stool.

Critical Thinking Exercise: Liver, Gallbladder, and Pancreas Disorders

Situation: A 40-year-old female, who is approximately 50 pounds overweight, seeks medical attention for chronic right upper quadrant (RUQ) abdominal pain. Based on her assessment and history, the primary care provider determines she most likely has cholecystitis.

1. List other risk factors, signs and symptoms, and the treatment for gallstones.

Diabetes Mellitus

Key Points

- Diabetes mellitus type 1 results from a destruction of beta cells in the pancreas, causing a complete lack of insulin production.
- Diabetes mellitus type 2 is related to insulin resistance at the cell level, with varying amounts of insulin production.
- Heredity is a risk factor for development of diabetes mellitus, type 2.
- Nutritional Committee of the Heart Association recommends increasing dietary fiber as one way to help lower blood sugar.

Overview

Diabetes mellitus is a metabolic disorder of energy balance with many causes and forms. A consistent sound diet is essential for diabetic control. A personalized nutrition plan that balances food, exercise, and insulin activity is necessary for successful management.

Types of Diabetes

- Primary forms
  - **Type 1, formerly known as insulin-dependent diabetes mellitus (IDDM)** develops rapidly and tends to be unstable. Persons are usually underweight and are prone to acidosis.
  - **Type 2, formerly known as non-insulin-dependent diabetes mellitus (NIDDM)** develops more insidiously and is milder and more stable. It occurs mainly in adults >40 years old and is associated with obesity.
- Secondary forms
  - **Gestational diabetes**—may be a result of the physiologic stress of pregnancy and the increased metabolic work that occurs.
  - **Diabetes associated with certain diseases**—may include pancreatic disease, alcoholism, or drugs.

Complications of Diabetes Mellitus

- Diabetic ketoacidosis (DKA)
- Hyper/hypoglycemia
- Infections
- Compromised healing

- Peripheral vascular disease
- Neuropathy
- Renal failure (Nephropathy)
- Accelerated cardiovascular and cerebrovascular disease
- Retinopathy

Causes

- Genetic factors
- Insulin resistance
- Lifestyle of excessive body fat, sedentary activity level, and stress
- Viral infection

Mild Hypoglycemia

As the blood sugar drops, the sympathetic nervous system is stimulated. The surge of adrenalin causes the following symptoms:

- Hunger
- Sweating
- Tremor
- Tachycardia
- Palpitation
- Irritability

Moderate Hypoglycemia

Impaired brain function can result from glucose deprivation. Signs of moderate hypoglycemia include:

- Headache
- Difficulty with concentration
- Confusion
- Slurred speech
- Visual changes
- Numbness
- Drowsiness

Severe Hypoglycemia

Hypoglycemic symptoms vary, depending on the individual, rate of drop, and usual baseline blood sugar. Another factor may be related to a decreased hormonal response to hypoglycemia, particularly in diabetics. Symptoms include:

- Difficulty arousing from sleep
- Seizure activity
- Disorientation or loss of consciousness

Clinical Manifestations of DKA

Without insulin, carbohydrates are not available to be used as energy. Instead, the body utilizes fat as an energy source. In uncontrolled diabetes mellitus, ketone production exceeds utilization. Clinical manifestations include:

- High serum glucose levels
- Occurance of glycosuria and ketonuria
- Drowsiness and lethargy
- Nausea and vomiting
- Hot and dry skin
- Fruity (acetone) odor to breath
- Deep and labored breathing
- Polyuria and weight loss
- Polydipsia
- Polyphagia
- Electrolyte imbalance

Diagnostic Assessment

- Self-monitoring blood glucose levels with home glucometer is an important part of maintaining a stable blood glucose level.
- Fasting-blood glucose is the level of glucose in the blood after an 8-hour fast; normal values are 70-110 mg/dL.
- Glycosylated hemoglobin (HgbA1c) sugar depends on the amount of glucose in bloodstream circulation over the RBC's 120-day life span. It is a reflection of the average blood sugar for 100-120 days before the test. Values are not affected by food intake, exercise, or stress.
- Lipid levels are important. High triglyceride level (>200 mg/dL) with an associated low level of high-density lipoprotein cholesterol (< 40 mg/dL) is generally found in persons with diabetes mellitus, type 2.

Goals of Nutritional Therapy

A dietitian should be consulted for individualizing meal plans according to the Exchange Lists for Meal Planning. The overall goal of nutritional therapy is to make changes in nutrition and exercise habits to improve metabolic control. Other goals are to:

- Maintain as near-normal blood glucose levels as possible by balancing food with either insulin or oral hypoglycemic agents, and by exercising.
- Achieve and maintain normal serum lipid levels.
- Provide adequate energy; maintain normal weight for adults, and normal growth and development for children.
- Prevent and treat acute complications of diabetes, hypoglycemia, and short-term illness; as well as long-term complications such as renal disease, cardiovascular, and cerebrovascular disease.

- Improve overall health through optimal nutrition.

Diet Therapy

- In this system using exchange lists, commonly used foods are grouped into 3 basic exchange lists according to approximately equal food values in specific portions.
- Exchange lists are based on current principals and recommendations for good diabetes control and health promotion.
  - The carbohydrate group is subdivided into lists of starch, fruit, milk, other carbohydrates, and vegetables.
  - The meat and meat substitutes group is sorted by fat content into very lean, lean, medium fat, and high fat.
  - The fat group is divided into monounsaturated, polyunsaturated, and saturated.
  - The total amount of food allowed for each day is divided into a specific number of exchanges from each group.
- Once the meal plan has been developed, it should be reviewed and possibly adjusted at least every 3-6 months.

Special Considerations

- Acute illness can contribute to increased blood sugar and liability of the levels. If dehydration and electrolyte imbalance occurs with infection or other illness, more serious complications, including DKA, can occur.
- Exercise affects the basal metabolic rate and consumption of energy forms. Modifying activity levels without dietary adjustment can result in abnormal blood sugar levels.

Critical Thinking Exercise: Diabetes Mellitus

1. Develop a teaching plan dealing with severe hypoglycemia in a client with diabetes mellitus, type 2. Include causes, signs and symptoms, and immediate treatment.

2. What client education information should be provided to the diabetic regarding the following:

Illness

Eating out

Stress

Cardiovascular Disorders

Key Points

- Cardiovascular disease leads to higher mortalilty rate than all forms of cancer combined and is the leading cause of death in the U.S..
- Heart disease results from several risk factors, mostly preventable ones.
- The silent risk factor for cardiac and vascular disorders without symptoms is essential hypertension.
- American Heart Association Dietary Guidelines: Revision 2000 issued a statement recommending increased consumption of fruits, vegetables, and whole grains; exercising regularly for at least 30 minutes; maintaining ideal weight; replacing saturated fats with fish and nuts, and limiting salt and alcohol intake.
- Fat accumulation around the midsection is associated with cardiovascular disease.

Overview

Many cardiovascular risk factors are associated with nutrition, and can be reduced by altering food habits and lifestyle. Dietary modifications include reducing total fats, particularly saturated fat, and cholesterol. There is a definite association between the amount and type of dietary fat, and an increased blood lipid level, including the triglyceride level. Adding more fiber in the diet, as well as engaging in regular and vigorous exercise in the daily routine, can help to lessen the risk for cardiovascular disease.

Coronary Artery Disease

The underlying pathological process in coronary artery disease (CAD) is atherosclerosis, which can cause vascular lesions and occlusions leading to angina pectoris.

- Assessment of total blood cholesterol is essential in evaluating CAD.

CAD Risk Classification		
Risk Class	Total Cholesterol	LDL Cholesterol
Desirable	200 mg/dL	<100 mg/dL
Borderline high	200-239 mg/dL	130-159 mg/dL
High	>240 mg/dL	160-189 mg/dL

- Dietary interventions for lowering and maintaining cholesterol should be implemented.
- Reduce total fat, saturated fat, and cholesterol.
- Guidelines should be 30% total kilocalories from fat, <7% saturated fat, and <300 mg cholesterol.
- Increase the amount of soluble fiber in the daily diet, including legumes, cereal grains, peas, beans, bananas, and many fruits and vegetables. Dietary fiber and soy product may reduce cholesterol absorption in the intestine.
- Some substances found in green tea are linked to the oxidation process, thereby reducing the risk of atherosclerosis.
- Certain types of pressed coffees may increase the LDL cholesterol in the body.
- Foods and dietary supplements containing higher doses of vitamin E may be useful in reducing cholesterol synthesis in the liver.
- Maintain a healthy weight within recommended guidelines for age, height, and body frame.
- Conservative intake of red wine is linked with reduced risk of cardiovascular disease due to the phenolic substances that act as antioxidants.
- High sugar diet may increase the risk of cardiovascular disease. The mechanism whereby an increase in insulin production causes lipoprotein synthesis in the liver.
- High dietary calcium intakes are likely to bind free fatty acid in the intestine, which reduces the fat absorption in the blood.

Hypertension

Hypertension is a risk factor for CAD. In about 95% of hypertensive cases, the cause is not known and is called primary or essential hypertension. Secondary hypertension is the term used when a cause is identified.

- First line of treatment is nonpharmacologic and is focused on lifestyle modifications.
- Weight reduction, minimal alcohol intake, regular physical exercise of at least 30 minutes at a time, 3-4 times per week, smoking cessation, and reduced sodium intake are all steps to take in controlling blood pressure.
- Average daily sodium intake is about 4-6 grams; only 500 mg is needed for normal bodily function. The American Heart Association guidelines recommend salt intake should be less than 2400 mg/day.
- Salt substitutes are used carefully, as each has a varying amount of sodium content.
- Sodium is "hidden" in many processed meats, dairy products, soups, marinades, condiments, and other foods.
- Niacin may cause vasodilatation in the client with hypertension.
- People who consume 5-9 servings of fruits and vegetables are less prone to heart disease, stroke, and hypertension.

- Eating foods rich in potassium, magnesium, and calcium can reduce blood pressure.
- Dietary intake of 2-4 servings/day of low-fat dairy products can also help to reduce blood pressure.

Myocardial Infarction

Cardiovascular disease is the most common cause of death in the U.S. The purpose of nutritional therapy is to reduce the workload of the heart and improve the vascular integrity and blood flow to vital organs.

- First 24 hours after cardiac injury, the diet is liquid and then progressed as tolerated.
- Small, frequent meals are better tolerated than large meals that increase myocardial oxygen demand.
- Caffeine-containing beverages and foods are limited to less than 4 servings/day to avoid myocardial stimulation.
- Foods and beverages should be of moderate temperature.
- Sodium, cholesterol, fat, and calories (if weight loss is needed) are controlled according to client's needs. Soy, dried beans, and legumes may be used as protein substitutes.
- Omega-3 fatty acids reduce the risk of blood clots that may cause a myocardial infarction.
- B6 (pyridoxine) and folic acid are recommended to reduce homocysteine levels.

Critical Thinking Exercise: Cardiovascular Disorders

1. In order to reduce coronary artery disease risk factors, a client who has an increased cholesterol level should initiate a diet to help lower blood cholesterol. For each component of the Food Guide Pyramid, list examples of foods to avoid or decrease in order to lower cholesterol.

Dietary Component	Foods to avoid
Milk and dairy products	
Meat, poultry, fish	
Eggs	
Breads, cereals, pasta, rice, dried beans	
Fruits and vegetables	
Fats and oils	

2. Clients who need to limit sodium intake require education about sodium that may be "hidden" in food. Food label reading should be included in a teaching plan. List at least 5 categories of foods that may contain large amounts of hidden sodium.

3. Using the Food Guide Pyramid, devise a plan for a client to eat "heart healthy." Give suggestions for each category.

Kidney Disease

Key Points

- Kidneys have three basic functions: Excretion of waste material, reabsorption of body constituents, and a metabolic hormonal role for regulation of fluid and electrolytes and acid-base balance.
- Renal disease interferes with the normal capacity of nephrons to regulate products of body metabolism.
- Short-term renal disease requires nutritional support for healing rather than dietary restrictions.
- Chronic renal failure requires nutrient modification according to individual disease status.
- Calcium, phosphorous, and vitamin D regulation occurs in the kidneys.
- The kidneys produce a hormone called erythropoietin that is important for the formation of red blood cells.

Overview

There are multiple nutritional components that need to be controlled with renal disease. Protein, phosphorus, sodium, and potassium are restricted, but kilocalories need to be at an adequately high level to prevent muscle protein from being broken down.

The primary roles of nutrition for the person with renal dysfunction are to control high blood pressure, minimize edema, decrease urinary albumin losses, prevent protein malnutrition, supply adequate energy, and slow the progress of the disease.

Acute Renal Failure (ARF)

Abrupt loss of renal function may or may not be accompanied by oliguria or anuria. Common causes of ARF are trauma, shock, and hemorrhage, as well as nephrotoxic medications or chemicals, septicemia, and strep infections.

- The stages of ARF include oliguric, diuretic, and recovery (may last 3-12 months).
- Nursing interventions include monitoring intake and output, daily weights, and meticulous skin care.
- Nutritionally, the client with kidney dysfunction may need to reduce protein, sodium, potassium, and fluid intake, depending on which stage of ARF. Foods high in potassium include dried beans, peas, soy, melons, and fruit.
- Be alert for constipation as a result of decreased intake of fluids, fresh fruits (increases potassium); bedrest, and medication side effects.

Chronic Renal Failure (CRF)

Chronic renal failure is a result of progressive, irreversible loss of kidney function. It may develop over a long time and progress to end stage renal disease. Common causes are glomerulonephritis, nephrosclerosis, obstructive disease, diabetes mellitus, lupus, and illicit use of analgesics and street drugs.

- Diet planning requires balancing needs for energy, protein, fats, phosphorus, potassium, sodium, vitamins, minerals, and fluids. Foods low in phosphorus include blueberries, strawberries, and raspberries.

- An exchange list, National Renal Diet, is used frequently as a guideline to manage CRF.

- Nutritional management also depends upon other therapies, such as hemodialysis or peritoneal dialysis.

- One goal of dietary management is to prevent uremic toxicity and delay the progression of renal disease.

- General signs and symptoms include: increased loss of renal function characterized by increased BUN/creatinine, change in urine color/output, weakness, shortness of breath, lethargy, fatigue, thirst, weight loss, diarrhea, vomiting, increased capillary fragility, muscular twitching, acidosis, and fetid breath.

Dialysis

Dialysis removes toxic substances from the blood and helps restore nutrients and metabolites to normal blood levels. A person with chronic renal failure (CRF) usually needs 2-3 treatments each week for 4-8 hours each.

- **Diet** is critical to maintain protein and kilocalorie balance, prevent dehydration or fluid overload, and maintain normal sodium and potassium, phosphate and calcium levels. Calcium carbonate may be given with meals to bind phosphate to foods.

- **Protein**: 1 g/kg lean body weight; 75% of this should consist of high biologic value, and very little milk because it adds more fluid and has increased sodium, phosphate, and potassium. A protein-rich diet helps to maintain muscle mass.

- **Kcalories**: 40 kcal/kg of carbohydrate (CHO). Simple CHO should be the bulk rather than complex types of sugars.

- **Water balance**: Limited to 400-500 cc/day plus an amount equal to urine output

- **Sodium**: Limited to 1000-2000 mg/day to control fluid retention

- **Potassium**: Restricted to 1500-2000 mg/day. Hyperkalemia may result in cardiac problems.

- **Vitamins**: Vitamin supplements are water-soluble since they are lost in dialysis.

- **Minerals**: Persons with renal failure requiring dialysis may experience excessive losses of copper via the exchange resin.

- **Saturated fat and cholesterol**: The Nutritional Committee of the American Heart Association recommends limiting dietary intake of saturated fat and cholesterol to reduce the risk of cardiovascular complications.

Renal Calculi

- Basic cause of kidney stones is unknown.
- Four major stones that form are: calcium, struvite, uric acid, and cystine.
- Formation of stones depends on several factors including low urine volume, high urine pH, and dietary habits.
- Each type of stone has its own medical and nutritional therapy.
- The best prevention is adequate fluid intake to keep the urine dilute, up to 2 L/day. Vitamin C supplements (>1000 mg/day) should be avoided, due to increased urinary oxalate excretion.
- **Uric acid stones** are formed as a by-product of purines. Limit foods high in purines such as sardines, gravies, organ meats, legumes, and whole grains. Dietary protein should not exceed 100 grams/day.
- **Calcium stones**: Current research indicates that limiting calcium intake is not needed since more stones form from oxalate. Oxalate is found in foods of plant origin, such as leafy green vegetables, rhubarb, spinach, and beets. Oxalate is an organic acid that depresses the absorption of calcium, thereby, causing increased excretion through the kidney.
- **Cystine stones** can be prevented by following the diet to avoid acidic urine and increased fluid intake.
- **Struvite stones** are not managed nutritionally. They occur more often in women with long-term antibiotic therapy and require surgical or ultrasonic removal.

Critical Thinking Exercise: Kidney Disease

1. Devise a teaching plan, including the best current advice for avoiding kidney stones.

2. Clients who have CRF need to reduce foods that are high in sodium. Make a list of obvious foods high in sodium, and a list of hidden sources of sodium.

Other Special Nutritional Problems

Key Points

- The overarching goal of nutrition therapy is to minimize nutritional complications of disease, to prevent muscle wasting, and to promote healing.
- Diet is one of the most important lifestyle factors in the etiology and prevention of cancer.
- Malnutrition is a common problem of HIV infection.
- Osteoporosis causes bone density reduction.

Overview

The conditions in this section deal with wasting diseases and malnutrition-related diseases, lack of calcium, and the effects of prolonged immobilization.

Cancer

- Environmental agents, genetic factors, and the functional level of the immune system relate to the development of cancer.
- Major treatments for cancer involve surgery, radiation, and chemotherapy.
- The disease process of cancer may cause anorexia, increased metabolism, and negative nitrogen balance.
- Systemic effects result in poor food intake, increased nutrient and energy needs, and more catabolism of body tissues.
- Nutritional needs for the cancer client include sufficient fuel for energy; a malnourished client needs 2500-3500 kcal/day.
- Dietary protein is increased to 100-150 g/day.
- Vitamin and mineral supplementation is needed.
- Adequate fluid intake is encouraged.
- Problems associated with nutritional management include anorexia, and early satiety; mouth ulcers; alteration in taste and decreased saliva, and gastrointestinal problems such as nausea, vomiting, and diarrhea.
- **Nutritional guidelines to cancer prevention:**
  - Adequate dietary fiber may lessen the risk of colon cancer.
  - Eliminate all tobacco to reduce the risk of lung cancer.
  - Peel, wash, or remove the outer leaves of fruit and vegetables, cut off excess fat.

- Thoroughly cook meats to reduce risks from environmental factors that may be carcinogenic.
- High intake of fruits and vegetables is linked to a lowered incidence of many different types of cancer.
- Intake of polyunsaturated and monounsaturated fats in fish and olive oils are presumed to be beneficial in lowering the risk of many types of cancer.
- High alcohol consumption is associated with various types of liver, pancreatic, and biliary cancers.
- Meat preparation with a smoking or pickling technique using nitrate-containing chemicals is potentially carcinogenic.
- Charcoal grilling with meat exposure to hydrocarbon substances may produce certain types of colon cancer.
- Excess body fat stimulates the production of estrogen and progesterone, which may intensify the growth of various cell types and may cause cancer, including breast, gallbladder, colon, prostate, uterine, and kidney.
- Familial link is a predominant association with many cancers (e.g., breast) requiring vigilant screening and healthy living practices.
- Calcium-rich diet is associated with a lower incidence of colon cancer because it binds free-fatty acids and bile salts in the lower gastrointestinal tract.
- Prolonged exposure to the sun is directly related to the occurrence of skin cancers.

- **Strategies to promote the nutritional status of the person with cancer, or receiving chemotherapy, or radiation therapy:**
  - Encourage the person to eat nutritious foods whether hungry or not.
  - Serve foods in an attractive manner to increase the appeal. Small, frequent servings are advised.
  - Provide a relaxing environment for meal or snack times.
  - A high-carbohydrate diet provides the needed energy without an extended feeling of satiety. Foods high in fat provide a feeling of fullness and remain in the stomach longer than carbohydrate foods.
  - Favorite foods should be offered when the client is feeling good to enhance the association with a pleasurable eating experience.
  - Offer short periods of rest during a meal. However, prolonged meal times can be tiring and reduce appetite.
  - Persons with diarrhea may benefit from a diet containing pectin. A low-residue diet helps reduce intestinal stimulation.
  - The client receiving immunosuppressant therapy may need to minimize exposure to microorganisms found on the outer layers of fresh fruit and vegetables. Peeling and thorough washing or cooking may be necessary. In some cases, fresh foods may may increase the risk for infection.
  - Foods should be soft and relatively bland when the person is experiencing nausea or has mouth sores. Sauces, gravies, and soups may be a desirable way to provide nutrients and calories without irritating the oral mucosa.

- To reduce metallic taste in foods, encourage the caregiver to prepare foods using plastic utensils. Serving utensils should also be non-metallic. Beef and pork produce a metallic or bitter taste.
- Encourage the use of straws when mouth ulcers are present. Meticulous oral care and possibly the use of local anesthetic for mouth sores may be necessary to prevent pain and allow sufficient oral intake.
- Liberal fluid intake is helpful to stimulate salivary secretions and moisture necessary for digestion, but liquids taken at mealtime can reduce the amount of food taken by filling the stomach.
- To combat dysphasia, the nurse may teach the client to inhale, swallow, and then exhale. Also, tilting of the head may help with swallowing. Avoiding sticky or lumpy food is advised.
- Cold foods are sometimes tolerated better than foods served hot. Sometimes the odor of foods during preparation can cause nausea. It may be better for the person with nausea, vomiting, and diarrhea to remain away from the food preparation area.
- Appetite-stimulating medication is not proven to be effective in the client with cancer or undergoing chemotherapy or radiation treatments.
- More information about cancer is available at: **http://www.cancer.org** and/or **http://www.cis.nci.nih.gov**.

Osteoporosis

- Osteoporosis is a condition in which bone density is reduced and the remaining bone is brittle and breaks easily.
- Causative factors include inadequate intake of calcium, poor absorption and metabolism of calcium, lack of physical exercise, immobility, and reduced estrogen production.
- Signs and symptoms include kyphosis or Dowager's hump of the vertebrae of the spine, decreased height, decreased bone density, and pathologic fractures.
- Primary sources of calcium rich foods that are encouraged include dairy and other milk- based products; nondairy sources such as green, leafy vegetables, small fish with bones, legumes, and tofu.
- Prevention is the key to osteoporosis and should begin at puberty, continuing throughout adolescence and adulthood.
- Begin calcium supplementation for women using hormone replacement therapy.

AIDS

- Autoimmune deficiency syndrome (AIDS) is a life-threatening disorder, caused by the retrovirus human immunodeficiency virus, which attacks T-cells and results in severe depression of immune function.
- Malnutrition is a common problem and is one of the causes of death in AIDS. Poor nutritional status leads to wasting and fever, and further aggravates the susceptibility to secondary infections.

- Decreased nutrient intake occurs because of physical symptoms such as anorexia, nausea, vomiting, and diarrhea; psychosocial symptoms may include depression, dementia, and restrictive regimens that may alter appetite.

- Diarrhea and malabsorption are prominent clinical problems in persons with AIDS. The nurse encourages dietary intake of the following foods to lessen the severity of diarrhea: applesauce, toast, hot cereal, rice, gelatin, bananas, crackers, broth, and potatoes. Liberal fluid intake is extremely important to prevent dehydration.

- Nutritional warning signs in HIV/AIDS clients include, rapid weight loss, gastrointestinal problems, inadequate intake, increased nutrient needs, food aversions, fad diets, and supplements.

- Clients need to be aware of potential health frauds related to unproved nutritional therapies.

- If the person with AIDS is unable to consume sufficient nutrients, calories and fluid, enteral feedings may be needed.

- More information about AIDS is available at: **http://www.aids.org**.

Prolonged Immobilization

- Bed rest can cause devastating atrophy and fatigue.

- Adequate protein intake is important to prevent further catabolism.

- Skin integrity may become compromised after just 24 hours of bed rest or 3 days of lying supine in bed.

- Immobilization causes a negative effect on muscle tone, bone calcium, plasma volumes, and gastric secretions.

- Glucose intolerance and shifts in body fluids and electrolytes may occur.

Critical Thinking Exercise: Other Special Nutritional Problems

1. Clients suffering from either cancer or AIDS may have diminished appetite, leading to malnutrition. For each of the following, list strategies for improving food intake.

    • Controlling nausea and vomiting

    • Increasing calories and protein

2. There are many causative factors of osteoporosis and decreased bone mineral density. Discuss at least two factors that can be modified with dietary management.

Critical Thinking Exercise Answer Keys

Situation: A client seeks assistance for weight control because she is "tired of being fat". Upon assessment, objective findings include 46-year-old female, 5′ 5″ tall, and 240 pounds. She also reports feeling out of control with her eating behavior and being disgusted with her physical appearance. The following questions relate to this client:

1. What are two of her major nursing diagnoses?

> **Alteration in nutrition: She is taking in more calories than energy expended as manifested by weighing more than recommended.**

> **Alteration in body image related to physical appearance of being obese as manifested by her verbalization of disgust.**

> **Alteration in thinking process related to body image disturbance as manifested by verbalization of being out of control with her eating behavior.**

2. In counseling this client, what are at least three characteristics of dietary principles that should be followed?

> **Set realistic goals.**

> **Reduce calories according to need.**

> **Assure nutritional adequacy of diet.**

> **Maintain culturally desirable foods.**

> **Readjust calories to maintain weight, after desired amount has been lost.**

3. What diseases might she be at risk for developing as a result of her obesity?

Obesity has been directly related to the development of Type 2 diabetes and hypertension, and secondarily related to the development of coronary artery disease and peripheral vascular disease.

4. For each of the foods in the following list, match them with the culture they are traditionally associated with:

Food		Culture
D	Bagel	A. Japanese
B	Baklava	B. Greek
A	Sushi	C. Native American
E	Bulgur	D. Jewish
C	Blue corn bread	E. Moslem

5. Devise a sample menu based on the Food Pyramid for a healthy adult female with an average weight. Develop the dietary plan based on approximately 1800 kcal/day and comprising of 50% of kcal from carbohydrate, 20% from protein, and 30% from fat sources.

Meal	Food	Serving
Breakfast	1 sliced orange 3/4 cup of a bran flake cereal with 1/2 cup non-fat milk 1/2 English muffin with 1 tsp soft margarine 6 oz vegetable juice Optional: coffee or tea	1 fruit 1 bread 1/2 dairy 1 bread 1 fat/sweet 1 vegetable
Lunch	Turkey sandwich with 2 slices of smoked turkey 2 slices of whole wheat bread 2 tsp mustard 2 lettuce leaves and tomato slices 1 Granny Smith apple 2 oatmeal raisin cookies Optional: diet soft drink	1 meat 2 bread 1 vegetable 1 fruit 2 fat/sweet

Meal	Food	Serving
Afternoon Snack	1 banana 1 Tbsp peanut butter 1/2 cup non-fat milk	1 fruit 1/2 meat 1/2 dairy
Dinner	5 oz grilled salmon with dill butter 1/2 cup rice 1/2 cup broccoli with 1tsp butter 1 dinner roll 1/2 cup non-fat milk 1/2 cup fruit sorbet	1 1/2 meat 1 fat 1 bread/grain 1 vegetable 1 fat 1 bread 1/2 dairy 1 fruit
Evening Snack	4 oz sharp cheddar cheese 4 whole wheat crackers	1 dairy 1 bread

Nutrient Content:

Bread and grains: 7 (recommended number of servings 6-11)

Fruit: 4 (recommended number of servings 2-4)

Vegetable: 3 (recommended number of servings 3-5)

Meat, fish, and poultry: 3 (recommended number of servings 2-3)

Dairy: 2 1/2 (recommended number of servings 2-3)

Sweet, fat oil: 5 (recommended using sparingly)

1. Compare and contrast the food-borne illness caused by *Escherichia* coli with that caused by *staphylococcus aureus*.

Food-borne Illness:	Staphylococcus Aureus	Escherichia Coli
Cause	Normally found on skin and may be transmitted to foods, especially salads, cream fillings, pies, milk, poultry, ham, and salad-based fillings.	Raw ground beef, maybe chicken, imported soft cheeses, and unsanitary handling of food and equipment.
Signs and Symptoms	Begins 2-6 hours after ingestion and includes nausea, vomiting, diarrhea, chills, and fever	Differ with each strain but may include bloody diarrhea, cramps, fever, chills, dehydration, and kidney failure
Prevention	Proper hand washing, refrigerating foods to decrease growth potential; not destroyed by heat, so cooking and boiling are not effective in making food safe to eat.	Proper hand washing, sanitary food handling, cook beef to well-done stage. Avoid cross- contamination between meat and other foods via cooking and preparation equipment and services.

2. Although various governmental agencies are responsible for food safety for consumers, we must also implement our own personal food safety plan. List at least four ways to ensure personal food safety.

- Hand washing is the number one priority.
- Cleanliness of equipment and surroundings is essential.
- Use hot soapy water with a disinfectant in it for cleaning.
- Use separate cutting boards for meat and vegetables.
- Food temperature should be either colder than 40°F or hotter than 140°F.
- Refrigerate cooked foods immediately after meals; do not cool at room temperature.
- Boil all home-canned foods for at least 10 minutes.
- Thoroughly cook all meat prior to consumption.
- Do not eat or even taste any uncooked foods prepared with raw eggs.
- After food shopping, refridgerate perishables as soon as possible.
- Never buy or use foods in bulging cans or with a dented or cracked lid or jar.

Digestion, Absorption, Metabolism, and Excretion Answer Key

1. Devise a chart that lists the three major nutrients and detail the digestive process, beginning in the mouth.

Carbohydrates	
Mouth	Starch-ptyalin-dextrins
Stomach	None
Small Intestine (pancreas)	Starch: amylase-maltose-sucrose
Intestine	Lactose: lactase-glucose & galactose Sucrose: sucrase-glucose & fructose Maltose: maltase-glucose & glucose

Protein	
Mouth	None
Stomach	Protein: pepsin-HCl acid-polypeptides
Small Intestine (pancreas)	Protein: polypeptides-trypsin-dipeptides Protein: polypeptides-chymotrypsin- dipeptides Polypeptides: dipeptides- carboxypeptidase-amino acids
Intestine	Polypeptides: dipeptides-aminopeptidase- amino acids Polypeptides: dipeptides-dipeptidase- amino acids

Fats	
Mouth	Fat-lipase: glycerides
Stomach	Tributyrin: tributyrinase-glycerol-fatty acids
Pancreas	Fat-lipase-glycerol Glycerides-di-mono Fatty acids-di-mono
Intestine	Fat: lipase-glycerol Glyceride: di-mono Fatty acids: di-mono
Liver and Gallbladder	Fat: bile-emulsified fat

Carbohydrates Answer Key

1. List the three categories of carbohydrates, common names for the appropriate ones, and examples of how they occur in natural food sources.

Carbohydrates	Common Name	Common Name
MONOSACCHARIDE		
Glucose	Blood sugar	Fruits, sweeteners
Fructose	Fruit sugar	Fruits, honey, syrup
Galactose		Part of lactose found in milk and sugar beets.
DISACCHARIDE		
Sucrose	Table sugar	Table sugar, sugar cane, sugar beets
Lactose	Milk sugar	Milk
Maltose	Malt sugar	Germinating grains
POLYSACCHARIDE		
Starch	Complex carbohydrate	Cereal, rice, grains, legumes, potato
Dietary fiber	Bulk	Whole grains, fruits, vegetables

1. Devise a simple plan for assisting a middle-aged male with high cholesterol and a family history of cardiovascular disease in gradually reducing his saturated fat and cholesterol food intake.

- Ask the client to keep a one-week food diary, listing all foods and beverages consumed. Encourage him to eat his normal foods and try not to alter them just because he is keeping track of them.

- After reading his diary, highlight foods with high saturated fat content and offer alternative suggestions.

- Encourage him to use lean cuts of meats, less red meat, and more poultry and seafood. Remove skin from chicken and trim visible fat. Avoid fat in cooking.

- Limit intake of eggs to 2-3 times each week; cook and serve them without added fat. Use egg whites freely, as well as egg substitutes.

- Select milk and dairy products that are 1% or 2%. Over a period of a few weeks reduce to non-fat products.

- Use seasonings, such as herbs, spices, lemon juice, onion, and fat-free broth, rather than cooking with fats.

- Remind him to schedule return visits to the primary care provider to monitor cholesterol levels. Explain how to read food labels for "hidden fat content."

Situation: An 18-year-old healthy female asks you about adopting the vegan style of eating. She is concerned about the health risks of eating meat, and also has strong beliefs about animal rights. Explain some of the benefits of a vegan diet, as well as some of the potential concerns.

---

1. Benefits of a vegan diet:

   Health benefits are similar to a low-fat, high-fiber diet.

   The diet may reduce the incidence of developing coronary artery disease (CAD), diabetes mellitus, type 2, gastrointestinal disorders, colon cancer, and hypertension.

   Cholesterol levels are typically lower.

   Some vegans tend to have a lower body weight due to the restriction of animal proteins that contain high caloric and high fat load, although others may replace protein with other types of dietary fat and, thus, not maintain a lean body type.

   A vegan diet is associated with less risk for food-borne diseases, such as E. coli or salmonella.

2. Concerns related to a vegan diet:

   The vegan diet may be lacking in essential amino acids.

   Vegans who do not comsume diary products may be lacking in vitamin D. Vitamin B$_{12}$ is most often found in animal-based foods. Strict vegan diets without vitamin B12 supplementation could lead to irrerversible nerve injury. As vitamin B12 is necessary for cell division and blood formation, persons consuming a plant-based diet are at risk for serious nutritional disorders. Childeren and pregnant or lactating women should be especially careful to receive sufficient amounts of vitamin B12.

   The vegan diet is also potentially lacking in iron, zinc, and calcium, as these are found in meat and milk products.

1. For each of the following vitamins, state the major function and a food source:

- Thiamine (B_1)

  B1 is a coenzyme in energy metabolism and nerve functioning. Lean pork, whole grains, legumes, nuts, and seeds are food sources.

- Niacin (B_3)

  B3 is a cofactor in energy metabolism. Food containing protein, enriched whole grains, peas, and nuts are food sources. Coffee also contains niacin and prevents pellagra in some cultures with low protein diets and high coffee intakes.

- Folate

  Folate is important in synthesis of amino acids and prevention of neural tube effects. Green leafy vegetables, ready-to-eat cereals, and fortified bread are food sources.

- Vitamin A (retinol)

  Vitamin A is important in vision and tissue strength and growth. Food sources include fish liver oils, liver, egg yolks, butter, and cream.

- Vitamin K

  Vitamin K is important for blood clotting. Green leafy vegetables are a good source of Vitamin K.

2. Vitamins are classified as either water-soluble or fat-soluble.

   Water-soluble vitamins are absorbed in the small intestine and passed into the bloodstream for circulation. Fat-soluble vitamins require bile for absorption to occur.

3. Pellagra is a niacin deficiency disorder characterized by specific symptoms. What physical manifestations can occur with pellagra?

Diarrhea

Dementia

Dermatitis

The dermatitis is a macular rash characteristically found on the bilateral sides of the face, feet, and hands, resembling gloves.

Large doses of niacin may cause a vasodilatation of the vascular system, which can result in a flushing effect. Toxicity does not result as an interference with other drugs.

1. Our bodies absorb calcium based on physiological need. Which factors tend to impact calcium absorption? Address factors such as high fiber diets, lactose, dietary fat, and sedentary lifestyle.

Bone cells, such as osteoclasts and osteoblasts, attract calcium and other substances to build or rebuild bone material.

Hormones, such as parathyroid hormone and calcitonin, regulate calcium and phosphorous metabolism in the body.

Vitamin D regulates tissue absorption of calcium for deposition in the bones and teeth.

Lactose is found naturally in milk and appears to increase calcium absorption.

Sunlight can potentiate the absorption of calcium.

High-protein intake increases calcium bioavailability if phosphorous is not consumed in equally high amounts.

Conservative intake of dietary fat makes calcium more accessible.

An active lifestyle and weight-bearing exercise leads to enhanced bone density.

High fiber moves food through the gastrointestinal tract too quickly, not allowing calcium to be absorbed.

Plant foods containing oxalates, bind with calcium making it unavailable to the body.

An alkaline environment decreases calcium solubility.

1. The body's requirement for water varies according to several factors. List and explain at least three of these factors.

Environmental temperature: Body water is lost as the environmental temperature increases, which helps maintain body temperature.

Physical activity: Increased physical activity may result in more water lost as perspiration, and more water required for increased metabolic demands of activities.

Functional losses such as vomiting and diarrhea will increase water loss.

Metabolic needs: 1 mL of water is needed to metabolize 1 kcal in the diet.

Age: An infant needs 1500 mL water/day, and the needs are critical because the total body weight of the infant is 70% water.

Situation: A 35-year-old primigravida is in her seventh month of pregnancy. Her total weight gain so far has been six pounds. Prior to becoming pregnant, she was approximately 40 pounds above ideal body weight. She is concerned about gaining too much weight during her pregnancy.

1. What nutritional information should you provide her?

   - A woman of normal pre-pregnant weight should gain between 20-35 pounds.
   - A woman who is above ideal body weight for height prior to pregnancy should gain approximately 15-25 pounds.
   - The normal weight gain pattern is 2-4 pounds in the first trimester, and then about one pound per week for the remainder of the pregnancy.
   - A severely restricted calorie diet is potentially harmful to the baby and the mother.
   - Calorie-restriced diets compromise energy and nutritional needs for the growth process.
   - This mother should eat at least the minimum number of servings from the Food Guide Pyramid on a daily basis.
   - Provide information about acceptable weight loss measures to be implemented after the birth of the baby.

1. Discuss the two hormones for lactation. Include the "let-down" reflex and inhibitors of that reflex.

> Prolactin is responsible for milk synthesis. As the baby latches and begins sucking after birth, a nerve impulse is sent to the hypothalamus. This, in turn, stimulates the anterior pituitary to secrete prolactin, which stimulates milk production.

> Oxytocin is also stimulated by infant sucking and is released from the posterior pituitary. This causes the milk glands to contract, thereby ejecting milk. This is called the "let- down" reflex and is usually felt as a tingling sensation in the mother's breast. This reflex may also be stimulated by hearing a baby cry, or by just thinking of her infant.

> The letdown reflex may be inhibited when the mother is unable to fully relax. Other inhibitors include being excessively tired or stressed, excessive alcohol or nicotine intake, or use of certain prescription drugs, such as anticholinergic agents.

2. When planning the diet of a woman who is breastfeeding, what recommendations would you include in your teaching?

> A reasonable approach is to recommend a diet that supplies at least 1800 kcal/day.

> The diet should be moderate in fat content.

> Encourage liberal fluid intake, especially water, of at least 2-3 liters/day.

> Include a variety of foods, such as milk, fruits and vegetables, and grains.

> Avoid caffeine-containing foods and beverages as they are passed through breast milk and can excite the central and autonomic nervous systems in the baby.

> Limit alcohol to one drink or less per day and not more often than twice a week.

> Instruct the breastfeeding mother to quit smoking because it lessens the production of breast milk.

> The lactating woman may want to avoid eating raw meat and fish because of the risk of toxoplasmosis, which could be transmitted to the infant through breast milk.

> Advise her not to follow an extreme caloric reduction diet, high-protein with low-fat diet, or any other fad or crash diet while breastfeeding. This could lead to impaired milk production and nutritional deficiency in the baby.

Situation: Parents of a 6-month-old infant want to know more about introducing solid foods to their child's diet.

1. What instruction might you give them?

Discuss the signs of developmental readiness for introduction of solid foods. The infant should be able to sit with support. The presence of an infantile protusion reflex can make sufficient feeding volume an arduous task.

The presence of an infantile protrusion reflex can make feeding volume an arduous task.

Foods should be introduced one at a time in small amounts to help identify any adverse reactions.

The first foods should be iron-fortified infant cereal, followed by strained fruits or vegetables.

Foods to avoid in the first year of life include honey (may cause botulism), hot dogs, grapes, hard candy, raw carrots, popcorn, nuts, peanut butter (choking), egg whites, and chocolate (allergies).

2. What nutritional information should be given to a mother who is breastfeeding twins or multiples?

Once pregnant weight is lost, the mother's weight loss/gain will indicate if she is eating enough. She should eat enough to satisfy hunger and focus on nutritious foods.

Breakfast is essential and should include high-protein food. The mother may want to supplement with one of the over-the-counter instant breakfast drinks.

Vegetables with a yogurt-based dip, cheese and crackers, sliced fruit, apples, and peanut butter are excellent snack choices and will provide extra calories.

Fluids should be increased to at least 80 ounces per day (240 mL/day), and should be consumed each time she nurses. Urine should be pale, rather than dark, as an indication of sufficient hydration. Avoid caffeine and alcohol-containing fluids.

A lactating woman should consume at least 500 calories extra per day for each nursing infant. These calories should come from a lean protein source.

1. Age-appropriate, nutritious snacks are important during childhood. List some healthy and attractive alternatives to refined sugar for a 9-year-old.

- Fruits washed, cut up, and stored in the refrigerator for easy access are healthy snacks; include apples, oranges, and melons
- Butter-free, salt-free popcorn
- Low-fat cheese and crackers
- Peanut butter sandwich with raisins
- English muffin
- Cottage cheese with fruit
- Fruit smoothies made with skim milk or fruit juices and protein powder supplement
- Yogurt or frozen yogurt

1. Anorexia is a psychological disorder characterized by self-imposed starvation. List the psychological and physical manifestations of anorexia.

Psychological	Physical
Distorted body image	Hair and nail changes
Obsession with body shape and size	Amenorrhea
Intense phobia of obesity	Fatigue
Hoards or hides food	Dehydration
Restricts own food intake but enjoys preparing	Electrolyte imbalances
food for others	Hypotension
Denies weight loss	Arrhythmias
Perfectionistic tendencies	Reproductive hormonal imbalances
Low self-esteem	Lanugo
Compulsive exercise	Loss of muscle mass and strength
	Vitamin, mineral, and protein deficiencies
	Mortality rate 5-10%

2. What recommendations would you make to an adolescent who has lactose intolerance in order to maintain an adequate calcium intake?

- **Drink orange juice or other juices fortified with extra calcium.**
- **Use tofu processed with calcium.**
- **Use lactose-free milk products.**
- **Drink rice milk.**
- **Apply lactose-free margarine.**
- **Take calcium supplements with primary care provider's advice.**
- **Ingest lactose tablets to aid digestion (with primary care provider's advice).**

1. The elderly person may be at increased risk for dehydration. Causes may range from senility and simply forgetting to drink, to consciously limiting fluids to avoid increased urination at night. List the common signs and symptoms of dehydration.

- Confusion
- Weakness, increased urinary sodium
- Hot, dry body
- Furrowed tongue
- Decreased skin turgor
- Rapid pulse

2. State some of the risk factors that may be associated with malnutrition in the elderly.

- Socioeconomic status, lack of finances
- Chewing and swallowing problems
- Digestive disturbances
- Lack of transportation to grocery store
- Impaired sense of taste and smell
- Multiple medications
- Diminished physical functioning
- Dementia and/or depression
- Anorexia
- Alcoholism

Food, Nutrient, and Drug Interaction Answer Key

1. Many medications have unpleasant side effects that are not caused by the illness. The side effects range from mild to severe. A common side effect of medications is gastrointestinal tract irritation and discomfort accompanied by nausea. List some nursing interventions that may be used to alleviate this particular side effect.

   For medicine that causes heartburn or indigestion, have the client sit up or stand after taking the medicine. A liberal water intake may help reduce the discomfort.

   Reduce intake of dietary fat, greasy foods, and foods with high citric acid.

   Reduce spicy foods, peppermint, chocolate, alcohol, pepper, and caffeine if these cause problems.

   Limit food intake in evenings to reduce reflux.

   Ensure adequate fluid volume; cold, carbonated, and clear liquids are easier to tolerate.

   Serve liquids after meals and only small amounts with meals to help with nausea.

1. Plan a sample menu for a client who is on a soft, low-fat diet. Include food selections for breakfast, lunch, and dinner.

   A soft, low-fat diet should consist of foods that have limited fiber and are easily digested. The low-fat portion should include a decrease in saturated fats and cholesterol.

   (Answers will vary, but may include a sample, such as the following:)
   Breakfast:
   Orange juice or apple juice
   Cream of wheat
   Poached or soft-boiled egg
   Toast
   Skim milk
   Coffee

   Lunch:
   Vegetable soup
   Crackers
   White meat turkey sandwich, texturized
   Lemon sherbet
   Skim milk or tea

   Dinner:
   Baked chicken with skin removed
   Baked potato
   Carrots (steamed)
   Peach slices
   Dinner roll
   Skim milk or tea

1. List and describe some of the nursing considerations for safely administering enteral tube feedings.

  • Temperature: Intermittent and bolus feedings should be administered at room temperature to decrease gastrointestinal side effects

  • Prevention of bacterial contamination: Use closed-feeding containers, change tubing administration set and bag daily, never add new formula to old formula, and do not hang feedings for more than 4-8 hours.

  • Prevention of aspiration: Check tube placement before feeding, elevated head of bed 30-45 degrees.

  • Patency of tube: Irrigate tube every 6-8 hours (continuous feed). For bolus or intermittent feeding, irrigate with 40-50 cc warm water after each feeding.

  • Medications: All should be in liquid form. Flush tubing before and after medicines with at least 20 cc water. Consult pharmacist before crushing or diluting any medications. Do not mix multiple medicines together to administer.

  • Monitoring: Confirm tube placement before each feeding; record urine glucose each shift until final rate and concentration are established; record gastric residuals every four hours, and record bowel movements, daily weights, intake and output, electrolytes, and chemistry profiles.

2. One of the most common complications of tube feeding is diarrhea. List two possible causes and the treatment for each.

  • Infection or bacterial contamination of formula: Confirm with cultures, limit bag hang time, change bag and tubing every 24 hours, and rinse after each bolus or before continuous feeds.

  • Malabsorption: Check for pancreatic insufficiency; change to low-fat, lactose-free, or elemental feedings; change to continuous feedings.

  • Bolus feeding or volume overload: Change to continuous feedings or temporarily decrease rate of feeding.

  • Medications: Evaluate type of medicine and their common side effects; change to fiber-containing formula; sorbitol-containing medicines may increase incidence of clostridium difficile.

  • Decreased bulk: Fiber-containing formulas may help normalize gastrointestinal transit time and bulk.

  • Protein-energy metabolism: Switch to isotonic formula and feed at slow rate.

1. Discuss clinical settings where parenteral nutrition

- Should be part of routine care:

    - Inability to absorb nutrients from the gastrointestinal tract (bowel resection, diseases of small intestine, radiation enteritis, severe diarrhea, intractable vomiting)
    - High dose cancer chemotherapy, radiation, and bone marrow transplantation
    - Moderate-to-severe pancreatitis accompanied by nonfunctional gastrointestinal tract

- Usually would be helpful:

    - Major surgery, total colectomy
    - Moderate trauma, 30%-50% body surface area burns, moderate pancreatitis, and neuro trauma
    - Inflammatory bowel disease
    - Hyperemesis gravidarum
    - Moderate malnutrition
    - Inflammatory adhesions with small bowel obstruction
    - Intensive cancer chemotherapy

1. Discuss a nursing care plan that deals with the responsibility for feeding clients with dysphagia. Include safe procedures and features of foods to be considered.

> Position the head upright, support with pillows if needed.

> Eliminate distractions so that the client can concentrate on the meal.

> Allow liquids after all food is cleared from the mouth.

> Encourage the client to eat small amounts and to chew well.

> Check for voice quality while eating; a wet or gurgled voice indicates food may be on vocal cords.

> The texture of the food can be modified: chopped, pureed, etc.

> The viscosity of liquids can be increased by thickening with commercial thickeners.

> Temperature extremes should be avoided, as they may cause coughing.

2. List at least four dietary treatment guidelines for peptic ulcer disease. Include the rationale for each.

> Eat five or six smaller meals rather than large ones to inhibit stomach distention.

> Avoid caffeine-containing beverages to decrease gastric secretions.

> Avoid alcohol in order to reduce damage to stomach lining.

> Avoid black pepper, chili powder, cloves, and nutmeg to decrease gastric secretions.

> Avoid aspirin to reduce irritation of stomach lining.

> Avoid cigarette smoking to promote healing of ulcer.

> Eat in a relaxed atmosphere to reduce stress.

> Avoid milk in order to prevent increased gastric acid secretion.

Liver, Gallbladder, and Pancreas Disorders Answer Key

Situation: A 40-year-old female, who is approximately 50 pounds overweight, seeks medical attention for chronic right upper quadrant (RUQ) abdominal pain. Based on her assessment and history, the primary care provider determines she most likely has cholecystitis.

1. List other risk factors, signs and symptoms, and the treatment for gallstones.

   Other risk factors for cholecystitis may include advanced age, female, obesity with high fat intake, hormonal imbalances, medications such as oral birth control pills, clofibrate, and cholestyramine, enzyme defects, and very low-calorie diets.

   Other signs and symptoms include mild, aching pain in the epigastric area that may increase and radiate to the RUQ and right scapular region, nausea, vomiting, tachycardia, diaphoresis. All symptoms are worse after a high-fat meal.

   When gallstones block the duct, it may cause inflammation that results in pain, tenderness, and fever. Fat intolerance may cause heartburn, flatulence, belching, epigastric heaviness, chronic upper abdominal pain, and nausea. Jaundice and steatorrhea may also be present.

   Recommended treatment is surgical removal of the gallbladder.

1. Develop a teaching plan dealing with severe hypoglycemia in a client with diabetes mellitus, type 2. Include causes, signs and symptoms, and immediate treatment.

> People with diabetes need to learn how to avoid hypoglycemia. The body utilizes glucose as a brain food and depends on a constant supply of it for metabolism and proper function. Prolonged lack of glucose can lead to permanent damage.

> Teaching Plan

> - Hypoglycemia can occur from too much insulin or from oral hypoglycemic medications, as a result of delayed meals, not eating enough CHO, or exercising too much without increasing food.
> - Signs and symptoms: perspiration; increased hunger, nervousness; skin is pale, cool, and clammy; mental confusion; tremor; weakness; headache; increased heart rate; blurred vision.
> - Blood glucose levels drop to below 70 mg/dL.
> - Onset is usually sudden and may be fatal if not treated.
> - Treatment: if client is conscious and can swallow, he/she should be given 15 grams of rapid-acting carbohydrates, such as 4 ounces of grape juice and graham crackers; recheck blood sugar in 15 minutes.
> - If person is unconscious, glucagon may be injected, IV solution of glucose administered, or a paste is applied to the gum line.
> - Diabetics should wear an ID bracelet to identify them as such, and should carry a convenient source of sugar with them at all times
> - After a hypoglycemic attack, a snack of complex CHO and proteins should be eaten.

2. What client education information should be provided to the diabetic regarding the following:

> Illness

> - During periods of illness, blood glucose levels may increase and diabetes control is more difficult.
> - Illness causes increased need for insulin, but there is a decrease in appetite and food intake.
> - Liquids and soft foods are better tolerated.
> - Monitor glucose at least every four hours before meals and adjust insulin accordingly.

- Contact primary care provider if illness lasts more than a few days.
- Increase fluids to prevent dehydration.

Eating out

- Choose restaurants that have appropriate food choices to make menu selection easier.
- Select simple foods without gravy or other sauces.
- Avoid sweets and alcoholic beverages.
- Try to apply the exchange list system whenever possible.
- Control the portions ordered.

Stress

- Physiologic or psychological stress alters blood sugar.
- Stress reducing techniques are taught.
- Relaxation techniques are practiced.

1. In order to reduce coronary artery disease risk factors, a client who has an increased cholesterol level should initiate a diet to help lower blood cholesterol. For each component of the Food Guide Pyramid, list examples of foods to avoid or decrease in order to lower cholesterol.

Dietary Component	Foods to avoid
Milk and dairy products	Whole milk, whole cheese, custard-style yogurt, non-dairy substitutes, cream cheese, sour cream; decrease 2% milk, creamed cottage cheese
Meat, poultry, fish	Organ meats, fatty and marbled meats, regular ground beef, goose, domestic duck, regular cold cuts, hot dogs, sausage, bacon, fried meat, canned meats; decrease peanut butter, nuts, shrimp, oysters
Eggs	Decrease egg yolks and use egg whites or substitutes
Breads, cereals, pasta, rice, dried beans	Egg noodles; decrease crackers, cakes, cookies, muffins
Fruits and vegetables	Coconut, fruits and vegetables in cream or sauces; decrease olives and avocados
Fats and oils	All fats, especially saturated fats, gravy, hydrogenated margarine, cocoa butter, cottonseed oil, coconut oil, palm oil; decrease mayonnaise

2. Clients who need to limit sodium intake require education about sodium that may be "hidden" in food. Food label reading should be included in a teaching plan. List at least 5 categories of foods that may contain large amounts of hidden sodium.

Hidden sodium may be found in any of the following categories of food:

- **Snacks such as corn chips, potato chips, peanuts**
- **Seasonings such as monosodium glutamate**
- **Soups, especially canned and dried mixes**
- **Sauces, including ketchup**

- Smoked meats and fish
- Sauerkraut and other pickled foods
- Sodium-processed lunchmeats
- Pre-prepared frozen meals

3. Using the Food Guide Pyramid, devise a plan for a client to eat "heart healthy." Give suggestions for each category.

- Heart healthy changes include eating a variety of foods each day
- Meats: Substitute dried beans or legumes as a main dish, trim fat from meats, remove skin from poultry, no frying, and buy tuna packed in water or olive oil.
- Milk: Gradually decrease from whole to 2% to skim.
- Cheeses: Choose low-fat cheese, 2-6 grams/fat/ounce.
- Ice cream: Use ice milk, yogurt, and sorbets.
- Eggs: Limit yolks to 3x /week.
- Fats and oils: Substitute soft margarine; limit lard and solid vegetable shortening.
- Vegetables: Eat raw or steamed, rather than fried, and fruits.
- Breads, cereals, and pasta: Use them as main dishes; use low-fat versions.

1. Devise a teaching plan, including the best current advice for avoiding kidney stones

   - **Increase fluid intake up to 2-3 liters per day to maintain more dilute urine.**
   - **Do not restrict dietary calcium.**
   - **Increase intake of fruits and vegetables (high in potassium).**
   - **Avoid organ meat, legumes, and whole grains to prevent uric acid stones.**
   - **Increase intake of complex carbohydrates.**
   - **Limit foods high in oxalate (spinach, rhubarb, leafy green vegetables, beets, nuts, chocolate, tea, strawberries) to prevent calcium stones .**
   - **Vitamin C supplements (>1000 mg/day) should be avoided because they increase urinary oxalate excretion.**

2. Clients who have CRF need to reduce foods that are high in sodium. Make a list of obvious foods high in sodium, and a list of hidden sources of sodium.

   Foods that are fairly obvious in their increased sodium content include:
   - **Condiments: pickles, olives, salted nuts, salad dressings, steak sauce, soy sauce, ketchup, mustard, seasoned salts**
   - **Breads/starches: crackers, potato chips, popcorn, pretzels**
   - **Meats/meat substitutes: cured, smoked, and processed meats, canned salmon and tuna, all cheeses, microwave foods, TV dinners, and peanut butter**
   - **Beverages: buttermilk, instant hot cocoa mix**
   - **Soups: canned, dehydrated, and bouillon**
   - **Vegetables: sauerkraut, pork and beans, canned tomatoes, vegetable juices**

   Clients need to be aware of sodium that is hidden in various dietary sources, so that appropriate choices may be made:
   - **Baking powder**
   - **Drinking water**
   - **Medication, such as antacids, laxatives, cough medicines, pain relievers**
   - **Food preservatives and additives to increase the shelf-life**
   - **Marinades and sauces**
   - **Beverages, particularly vegetable juice and soft drinks**

1. Clients suffering from either cancer or AIDS may have diminished appetite, leading to malnutrition. For each of the following, list strategies for improving food intake.

   - Controlling nausea and vomiting

     - Eat small frequent meals
     - Eat dry foods with fluids in between
     - Cold foods and salty foods are better tolerated
     - Avoid fatty or sweet foods
     - Do not lie down immediately after eating
     - If vomiting occurs, replace fluids with juices; broth; ginger ale, and sports drinks

   - Increasing calories and protein

     - Fortify foods with high calorie condiments and dressings
     - Add extra ingredients, such as dry milk and cream
     - Use supplemental protein supplements
     - Eat more when the appetite is good
     - If mouth is sore, use soft foods, and avoid hot or cold temperature extremes

2. There are many causative factors of osteoporosis and decreased bone mineral density. Discuss at least two factors that can be modified with dietary management.

   - Nutrition/calcium intake: It is important to take in the RDA, particularly during the growth years and in post menopausal years of bone mineralization loss.
   - Alcohol: Long-term, excessive intake of alcohol may reduce bone density and may directly depress bone formation.
   - Smoking: Smokers tend to have less bone density and lose more bone mineralization.
   - Caffeine: There is a link between caffeine use and urinary excretion of calcium.
   - Sedentary lifestyle: Physical activity enhances calcium absorption and helps to maintain bone mineralization.

Dudek, S. G. (2006). *Nutrition Essentials for Nursing Practice* (5th ed.). Philadelphia: Lippencott Williams and Wilkins Publishers.

Grodner, M., Long, S., & DeYoung, S. (2004). *Foundations and clinical applications of nutrition: A nursing approach* (3rd ed.). St. Louis, MO: W.B. Mosby.

Kessel, M., & Wardlaw, G. M. (2002). *Perspectives in nutrition* (5th ed.). New York: McGraw Hill.

Mitchell, M.K. (2003). *Nutrition Across the Lifespan* (2nd ed.). Philadelphia: W.B Saunders Company.

Peckenpaugh, N. J., & Poleman, C. M. (2003). *Nutrition: Essentials and diet therapy* (9th ed.). Philadelphia: W. B. Saunders Company.

Wardlaw, G. M., & Kessel, M. (2002). *Perspectives in nutrition* (5th ed.). St. Louis, MO: McGraw Hill.

Williams, S. R. (2005). *Basic nutrition and diet therapy* (12th ed.). St. Louis, MO: Mosby-Year Book, Inc.